More Praise for *The Art of Dying Well*

"In plain English and with plenty of true stories to illustrate her advice, Katy Butler provides a brilliant map for living well through old age and getting from the health system what you want and need, while avoiding what you don't. Armed with this superb book, you can take back control of how you live before you die."

—Diane E. Meier, MD, director,
Center to Advance Palliative Care

"Katy Butler has given us a much-needed GPS for navigating aging and death. *The Art of Dying Well* is a warm, wise, and straightforward guide, hugely helpful to anyone—everyone—who will go through the complex journey to the end of life."

—Ellen Goodman, founder, The Conversation Project

"I wish every one of my patients would read this book—it is like having a wise friend explaining exactly what you need to know about coping with aging or living with a serious illness. It's not only about dying—it's about getting what you need from your medical care, including all the insider stuff your doctors and nurses don't always want to say. We can all learn from Katy Butler—especially doctors—about how to talk to each other more clearly and kindly about decisions that matter."

—Anthony Back, MD, Medical Oncology and
Palliative Medicine, codirector, Cambia Palliative
Care Center of Excellence, University of Washington

ALSO BY KATY BUTLER

Knocking on Heaven's Door

The Art

–of–

Dying Well

A Practical Guide to a Good End of Life

KATY BUTLER

Scribner

NEW YORK · LONDON · TORONTO · SYDNEY · NEW DELHI

SCRIBNER
An Imprint of Simon & Schuster, Inc.
1230 Avenue of the Americas
New York, NY 10020

First Scribner hardcover edition February 2019

SCRIBNER and design are registered trademarks of The Gale Group, Inc., used under license by Simon & Schuster, Inc., the publisher of this work.

For information about special discounts for bulk purchases, please contact Simon & Schuster Special Sales at 1-866-506-1949 or business@simonandschuster.com.

The Simon & Schuster Speakers Bureau can bring authors to your live event. For more information or to book an event, contact the Simon & Schuster Speakers Bureau at 1-866-248-3049 or visit our website at www.simonspeakers.com.

Manufactured in the United States of America

5   7   9   10   8   6

Library of Congress Cataloging-in-Publication Data

Names: Butler, Katy, 1949– author.
Title: The art of dying well : a practical guide to a good end of life / by Katy Butler.
Description: First Scribner hardcover edition. | New York : Scribner, 2019.
Identifiers: LCCN 2018037020 | ISBN 9781501135316 (hardback) | ISBN 9781501135477 (paperback)
Subjects: LCSH: Terminal care. | Death. | BISAC: SELF-HELP / Death, Grief, Bereavement. | MEDICAL / Terminal Care. | BIOGRAPHY & AUTOBIOGRAPHY / Personal Memoirs.
Classification: LCC R726.8 .B882 2019 | DDC 616.02/9–dc23
LC record available at https://lccn.loc.gov_2018037020

ISBN 978-1-5011-3531-6
ISBN 978-1-5011-3532-3 (ebook)

TO BRIAN DONOHUE

anam cara

Author's Note

This is a work of nonfiction and its stories are based primarily on interviews with direct participants. There are no composite characters, rejiggered timelines, made up quotes, or invented scenes. When names have been changed, it is disclosed in the notes.

Contents

INTRODUCTION

The Lost Art of Dying

1

CHAPTER 1

Resilience

The Wake-Up Call • Building Reserves • Finding Allies
in Preventive Medicine • Weighing Medical Risks •
Getting to Know the Neighbors • Knowing Your
Medical Rights • Caring for the Soul

11

CHAPTER 2

Slowing Down

When Less Is More • Simplifying Daily Life • Finding
Allies in Slow Medicine, Geriatrics, and a Good HMO •
Reviewing Medications • Reducing Screenings •
Making Peace with Loss

35

CHAPTER 3

Adaptation

A Moment of Truth • Mapping the Future and Making
Plans • Finding Allies in Occupational and Physical
Therapy • Disaster-Proofing Daily Life • Making a Move •
Practicing Interdependence • Being an Example

53

CHAPTER 4
Awareness of Mortality
The Art of Honest Hope • Talking to Your Doctor •
Understanding the Trajectory of Your Illness • Preparing
the Family • Finding Allies in Palliative Care • Reflecting
on What Gives Your Life Meaning• Staying in Charge •
Thinking Creatively • Redefining Hope

75

CHAPTER 5
House of Cards
If Only Someone Had Warned Us • Recognizing
Frailty • Avoiding the Hospital • Finding Allies in
House Call Programs • Upgrading Advance Directives •
Coping with Dementia • Shifting to Comfort Care •
Enjoying Your Red Velvet Cake

105

CHAPTER 6
Preparing for a Good Death
Making Good Use of the Time You Have Left • Finding
Allies in Hospice • Next Steps • Settling Your Affairs •
Choosing the Time of Death • Loving, Thanking, and
Forgiving • Getting Help from Your Tribe

135

CHAPTER 7
Active Dying
The Tree Needs to Come Down • This Is What Dying
Looks Like • Preparing for a Home Death • Preparing in
a Nursing Home • Giving Care • The Final Hours •
Humanizing a Hospital Death • Improvising Rites of
Passage • Welcoming Mystery • Saying Goodbye

161

CONCLUSION
Toward a New Art of Dying
195

Glossary
213

Resources
231

Notes
243

Acknowledgments
257

Permissions
261

Index
263

I Worried

I worried a lot. Will the garden grow, will the rivers
flow in the right direction, will the earth turn
as it was taught, and if not how shall
I correct it?

Was I right, was I wrong, will I be forgiven,
can I do better?

Will I ever be able to sing, even the sparrows
can do it and I am, well,
hopeless.

Is my eyesight fading or am I just imagining it,
am I going to get rheumatism,
lockjaw, dementia?

Finally I saw that worrying had come to nothing.
And gave it up. And took my old body
and went out into the morning,
and sang.

—MARY OLIVER

The Lost Art of Dying

To our ancestors, death was no secret. They knew what dying looked like. They knew how to sit at a deathbed. They had customs and books to guide them—and a great deal of practice.

Consider, for instance, death's presence in the lives of my great-great-great-grandparents, Philippa Norman, a household servant, and John Butler, a brush- and bellows-maker. Poor Quakers, they married in Bristol, England, in 1820 and had four children, two of whom died before their second birthdays.

In hopes of starting a new life, John sailed to New York in 1827 on the ship *Cosmo*; Philippa and their surviving son and daughter followed the next year. In their rented rooms there, Philippa gave birth to a stillborn son and later sat at John's bedside as he died of tuberculosis, now preventable with vaccines and treatable with antibiotics.

Widowed at thirty-six, Philippa sailed back to Bristol. There she nursed her beloved daughter Harriet as she, too, died of tuberculosis, in her early twenties. Only one of Philippa's five children—her son Philip—would live long enough to marry and have children of his own. And one of those children, Philip's favorite daughter Mary, died in 1869 at the age of thirteen when typhoid fever swept through her Quaker boarding school.

If you look closely at your own family tree, you will probably discover similar stories.

People in developed countries now inhabit a changed world, one in which dying has largely been pushed into the upper reaches of the life span. There it awaits us, often in shapes our ancestors would not recognize. To have postponed it so long often means we meet it—as my family did—unprepared.

My father enjoyed a vigorous old age until he was seventy-nine. Then one fall morning, he came up from his basement study, put on the kettle, had a devastating stroke, and began a process of slow-motion dying. My mother and I, who would become his caregivers, had little sense of the terrain ahead, and even less familiarity with the bewildering subculture of modern medicine.

As I described in my prior book, *Knocking on Heaven's Door: The Path to a Better Way of Death*, we were ignorant of medicine's limits, and the harm it can do, when it approaches an aging human being in the same way as it does the bodies of the young.

Two years later, my father was given a pacemaker to correct his slow heartbeat. This tiny electronic device made him, as he put it, "live too long" by forcing his heart to outlive his brain. He spent his last six and a half years dependent on my exhausted mother, descending step-by-step into deafness, near-blindness, dementia, and misery. Close to the end, my mother and I embarked on a modern rite of passage: asking his doctors to deactivate a medical technology capable of preventing his death without restoring him to a decent life. His doctors refused.

My father finally died quietly, over the course of five days, in a hospice bed, with his pacemaker still ticking. My mother and I had quite consciously decided not to allow his pneumonia (once called "the old man's friend") to be treated with antibiotics. I was fifty-nine then, and had never before sat at a deathbed. Perhaps it was my great good luck to have been shielded for so long. But it was also my burden. During my father's last days, I sat alone for hours in that clean but generic hospice room, holding his hand, bereft of the "habits of the heart," long practiced by my ancestors, that could have made his dying a more bearable and sacred rite of passage.

We live in a time when advanced medicine wards off death far better than it helps us prepare for peaceful ones. We feel the loss. Many of us hunger to restore a sense of ceremony, community, and yes, even beauty, to our final passage. We want more than pain control and a clean bed. We hope to die well.

TOWARD A NEW ART OF DYING

In the mid-1400s, when the Black Death was still fresh in cultural memory, an unnamed Catholic monk wrote a medieval death manual called *Ars Moriendi,* or *The Art of Dying.* Written in Latin and illustrated with woodcuts, it taught the dying, and those who loved them, how to navigate the physical and spiritual trials of the deathbed. One of the West's first self-help books, it went through sixty-five editions before 1500, and it was translated into all the major languages of Europe.

In each woodcut, a dying man or woman lies in bed, attended by friends, spouses, angels, and sometimes a doctor, servant, or favorite hound. Beneath the bed are demons, urging the gravely ill person to give in to one of five "temptations" standing in the way of dying in peace. Those were lack of faith, despair, impatience, spiritual pride, and what the monk called "avarice"—not wanting to say goodbye to the cherished things and people of the world. We no longer call them "temptations," but these emotions—fear, remorse, wanting to die quickly, and not wanting to die at all—are familiar to most who have sat at a deathbed.

The antidote, counseled the *Ars Moriendi,* was not to fight bodily death by medical means, but to care for the soul. The manuals encouraged the dying to confess their regrets and fears to their friends, and even provided scripts for attendants to recite, to reassure dying people of God's forgiveness and mercy. The dying were then invited to "commend their souls" into the hands of God and to relax into a state of grace. The soul, pictured in the woodcuts as a tiny human being, would leave the body and fly to heaven in the company of an army of angels. Sometimes a roof tile would be loosened to ease its escape.

In the *Ars Moriendi*, the dying were not passive patients, but the lead actors in their lives' final, most important drama. Even on their deathbed, even in pain, they had choices and moral agency. Their dying was domestic and communal, as sacred and as familiar as a baptism or a wedding.

Over the next four centuries, emerging religions wrote their own versions of *The Art of Dying*. Anglicans consulted *The Waye of Dying Well*, while Quakers like my ancestors studied accounts of the stoic deaths of their devout fellows in *Piety Promoted: In Brief Memorials and Dying Expressions of Some of the Society of Friends, Commonly Called Quakers*. That book, repeatedly updated with new death stories, was still in print in 1828 when my ancestor John Butler died in New York.

In those days, dying happened at home under the care of family and friends. It usually took days or weeks—not years. Children, dogs, and even neighbors would gather at the bedside to say their farewells. Prayers were spoken. A priest might visit. Candles were lit. When death came, the local church bell would toll, informing the entire neighborhood.

After the final breath, relatives or volunteers would ceremonially wash and dress the body, a tradition observed in nearly all cultures and religions. In Ireland, a wake, a party blending the holy and the worldly, would be held over the coffin to celebrate and say goodbye to the dead and to help the living make the transition back toward life.

In America today, church bells no longer toll when someone dies. In hospitals and nursing homes, the dead are usually zipped into body bags and gurneyed out back elevators, as if death itself was a frightening and shameful failure.

The demons under the bed have taken new forms.

Even though more than three-quarters of Americans still hope to die at home, fewer than a third of us do so; the rest of us die in hospitals, nursing homes, or other institutions. Nearly a third spend time in an intensive care unit in the month before they die, and 17 percent of Americans die in an ICU.

In antiseptic rooms, hospital protocols replace ancient rites. The dying often can't say their last words, because they're sunk in chemical twilights or have tubes down their throats. Relatives pace the halls, drinking bad coffee from vending machines, often shocked to hear for the first time, in a drab conference room, that someone they love is so close to dying. Nurses and doctors sometimes use the word "torture" to describe what happens in the ICU when a member of the medical team, or of the family, refuses to accept the coming of death. Treatment doesn't stop until someone gathers the courage to say "no."

The modern custom of reducing dying to a medical procedure, and stripping it of dignity and humanity, is intensifying in most parts of the United States. Resistance—inside and outside hospitals—is growing in equal measure. Many people yearn to reclaim the power to shape how they (and those they love) die, but aren't sure how to go about it.

There is a way to a peaceful, empowered, humane death, even in an era of high-technology medicine. It begins long before the final panicked trip to the emergency room. It requires navigating—over years, not days—a medical system poorly structured to meet the needs of aging people, and of people of any age coping with a prolonged or incurable illness.

That system pours its money, energy, and time into saving lives, curing the curable, and fixing the fixable. In its division of labor, it looks much like an auto assembly line. Each specialist works on a single vital organ and puts the body back on the conveyor belt. Every year, this "fast medicine" track saves countless victims of violence, car accidents, and heart attacks. In a crisis, it works very well.

But when people confront an incurable condition that can be managed, but not fixed, the conveyor belt offers more and more procedures that pose greater and greater risks. The body becomes globally fragile. Now, fixing things organ by organ, and assuming that living as long as possible is every person's paramount goal, can create obstacles to living well despite imperfect health, and to dying in peace.

Prolonging the life of the body is only one of medicine's traditional missions. The others are: preventing disease; restoring and preserving function; relieving suffering; and attending the dying. As we age, these "quality of life" goals grow in importance. But conveyor belt medicine, which absorbs the bulk of our insurance dollars, has largely forgotten how to address them. It rewards *cure* far better than *care*. It often does things *to* people, not *for* them, and turns them into passive bystanders to their own health. It shuttles the sick and fragile from specialist to specialist, and from doctor's office to emergency room and back again. The older or frailer we get, the wider the gap is likely to grow between the treatments fast medicine offers and the thoughtful, time-consuming gentle, coordinated care we need most.

In the years I've spent listening to hundreds of people's stories of good and difficult declines and deaths, I've learned one thing: people who are willing to contemplate their aging, vulnerability, and mortality often live better lives in old age and illness, and experience better deaths, than those who don't.

They keep shaping lives of comfort, joy, and meaning, even as their bodies decline. They get clear-eyed about the trajectory of their illnesses, so they can plan. They regard their doctors as their consultants, not their bosses. They seek out medical allies who help them thrive, even in the face of disappointment and adversity, and they prepare for a good death. They enroll in hospice earlier, and often feel and function better—and sometimes even live longer—than those who pursue maximum treatment. They make peace with the coming of death, and seize the time to forgive, to apologize, and to thank those they love. They rethink the meaning of "hope." And they often die with less physical suffering, and just as much attention to the sacred, as our ancestors did.

But those who give up their power, hoping only to postpone death and never facing where things are heading, often ride the conveyor belt to its ultimate destination: a high-tech hospital room. And there, in a place where success is defined as *not dying,* they die.

This is not what most of us want. A 2017 poll, asking people to think about the ends of their lives, found that only one-quarter wanted to live as long as possible, no matter what. The rest cared much more about the quality of their lives and deaths: not burdening their families, being at peace spiritually, dying at home, and dying comfortably. If you are among those three-quarters, this book is for you. It is intended to help you remain your life's lead actor from the first inklings of old age or serious diagnosis, all the way to the end. It can be done.

There is a reform movement dedicated to restoring meaning and dignity to end-of-life care. Outside medicine, it is reflected in the grassroots meetups called "Death Cafes" and in the success of best-sellers like Atul Gawande's *Being Mortal,* Barbara Ehrenreich's *Natural Causes,* and Paul Kalanithi's *When Breath Becomes Air.* Each book, each meeting, each honest conversation is ripping away the shame and secrecy that has, in the past century, made us more terrified of death, and more unequipped for it, than we need be. Within the health care system, this budding movement goes by many names, including value-based medicine, shared medical decision-making, Slow Medicine, and patient-centered care. Its pioneers include many brave, emotionally skilled oncologists and nurses who have never forgotten that their patients' needs and desires should come first, and others trained in primary care, geriatrics, occupational and physical therapy, palliative care, and hospice. All can coach you in the art of living well long before they help you die well.

HOW THIS BOOK IS ORGANIZED

This is a step-by-step guide to remaining as healthy and happy as possible, and as medically informed and unafraid, through the predictable health stages of later life, from vigorous old age to final breath. I have devoted one chapter to each stage: *Resilience, Slowing Down, Adaptation, Awareness of Mortality, House of Cards, Preparing for a Good Death,* and *Active Dying.* The goal of each chapter is to help you thrive and keep you on a path to a good end of life—however *you* define it.

Each chapter will suggest ways to step off the conveyor belt of fast medicine when it no longer serves you, and to find medical allies focused on what matters most to you, be it staying functional, controlling your physical pain, or emotionally supporting you and those whom you love. I hope its true stories will help you understand where each medical choice is likely to lead. Stage by stage, year by year, and decade by decade, you will probably lean more and more on gentle approaches that support a good quality of life, even as it winds down. The balance you strike, and how and when you shift, is up to you.

This book will, I hope, wherever you are on the journey from birth to death, give a rough sense of the time that remains, and empower you to stay in charge of a changing relationship to medicine. This is the best way I know to make room for your own versions of the rites of passage that our ancestors so prized. The temple of the sacred will be built upon a foundation of the mundane.

It is my deep hope that you will be peaceful and at ease at the moment of your death. That you may be safe, well supported, and free from fear long before that day comes. That you have what you need—emotionally, medically, spiritually, and practically—to live fully until your last breath. That you and those who love you may be held in the arms of a loving community and a competent medical team.

That is my desire. I wish this book could guarantee you a vigorous old age, a short decline, and a swift, painless death at home, surrounded by those who love you. But as the eighteenth-century German physician Zacharias Schultz wrote, people have long wished for "a gentle, mild and sweet" death, and feared one that is "arduous, terrible and hard." This, he said, had long been the focus of people's pious prayers, as well as their pleas to their doctors. Now more than ever, the way we die can be uncertain, ambiguous, attenuated, and prolonged. No matter how bravely we adapt to loss and how cannily we navigate our fragmented health system, things will not always go as we imagine. And yet if we want to keep shaping our lives all the way to the end, it helps to imagine, to choose, and to plan.

I am not suggesting we create a new Art of Dying to make death somehow perfect. Perfection is not a goal of art; it is an ambition of technology and science. Arts are improvised out of the limited, imperfect materials at hand. A modern Art of Dying will not make the end of every life painless, but it can make it bearable, shared, and even, in its own way, beautiful. Here is a compass and the beginnings of a map.

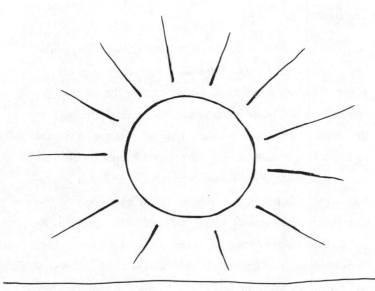

CHAPTER 1

Resilience

The Wake-Up Call • Building Reserves
Finding Allies in Preventive Medicine • Weighing Medical Risks
Getting to Know the Neighbors • Knowing Your Medical Rights
Caring for the Soul

The River Grows Wider

Some old people are oppressed by the fear of death. . . . The best way to overcome it is to make your interests gradually wider and more impersonal, until bit by bit the walls of the ego recede, and your life becomes increasingly merged in the universal life. An individual human existence should be like a river: small at first, narrowly contained within its banks, and rushing passionately past rocks and over waterfalls. Gradually the river grows wider, the banks recede, the waters flow more quietly, and in the end, without any visible break, they become merged in the sea, and painlessly lose their individual being. [Those] who can see life in this way will not suffer from the fear of death, since the things [they care] for will continue.

—BERTRAND RUSSELL

You may find this chapter useful if you recognize yourself in some of the following statements:

- You easily blew out all the candles on your fiftieth or sixtieth birthday cake.
- Aches, pains, and health problems are annoying but not limiting. You pay your own bills, make your own medical decisions, and generally enjoy life.
- You wonder why they make the numbers on credit cards so small and fuzzy.
- Your hair is thinning in familiar places and sprouting in strange ones.
- You misplace keys—and names. You're not crazy about technology updates.
- A late night blows a hole in the next day. Sometimes you're in bed by nine. You've discovered naps.
- Getting in shape takes longer, and the results are less impressive. You injure more easily and recover more slowly.
- Some friends have died. You find obituaries interesting.
- You sometimes sense that your time on earth is limited and precious.

THE WAKE-UP CALL

Doug von Koss was born in the Depression and raised on the banks of the Mississippi River in a houseboat his father built from salvaged lumber. In the 1960s he settled in San Francisco, where he and his wife, Clydene, raised their son and daughter. He made his living as a stagehand, theater carpenter, light board operator, and set dresser for films like George Lucas's *Return of the Jedi.* He's now eighty-five, tall, elegant, and commanding. Widowed for a decade, he lived in a neat, rented bungalow on a hilly San Francisco street.

In his fifties, while he was working as prop master for the San Francisco Opera, he led a workshop in mask making at a men's conference in the redwoods of northern California. The men, who'd just met, nervously labored over their masks in silence, with pinched faces and little joy. The poet Robert Bly, one of the conference organizers, nudged Doug's arm and said, "Get them singing." Doug drew the men outside. After twenty minutes of belting out camp songs under the redwoods, the men loosened up, started talking with each other, and returned to sculpting their masks with abandon. Ever since, Doug has been flying around the country, helping groups build community by leading them in traditional songs, chants, and poems that he's gathered from cultures around the world.

Not long after his seventy-ninth birthday, Doug found the steps up to his front door growing steeper by the day. At first, he brushed off his fatigue and breathlessness as normal aging. Then one midsummer afternoon, as he was pushing a shopping cart through the supermarket, he felt light-headed, dizzy, and short of breath. He trundled over to the one place where he could sit down: the do-it-yourself blood pressure machine near the pharmacy. He doesn't remember now whether his reading was too high or too low, only that it wasn't good.

The next morning in a medical building downtown, his doctor stopped in the middle of recording Doug's electrocardiogram and called an ambulance. EMTs took Doug down the elevator on a gurney. Twenty-four hours later, in a cardiac lab at a nearby hospital, doctors inserted a small tubular metal cage called a stent into an artery leading to the heart's largest blood vessel. "One of the main vessels was plugged," Doug said. "I could have gone belly up." He'd been millimeters from a heart attack.

The stent pushed aside a clump of fatty plaque, propped open the artery walls, and increased the flow of oxygen-rich blood to Doug's heart, body, and brain. He found it almost instantly easier to climb his front stairs. "Life became incredibly sweet," he remembered. "I could stop and look at a tree, look at a flower, and really *see* it. I felt really alive, and at the same time very fragile."

The stent, he sensed, was a temporary reprieve. Why, he wondered, had fat, cholesterol, and calcium congealed in his arteries? He didn't smoke or drink, never touched bacon, and rode his bike in Golden Gate Park three times a week. "But I got the message," he said. *"Pay more attention, Doug. There's a line between disease and optimum wellness, and you're sliding into disease."*

His hospital offered a four-month program of intensive cardiac rehabilitation, paid for by Medicare. Three times a week at a rehab center, he strapped on a heart monitor and pedaled a stationary bicycle while a physical therapist helped him gradually increase his heart rate. A dietician nudged him toward the Mediterranean Diet—less meat, dairy, sugar, and packaged foods; more vegetables, whole grains, olive oil, fish, and fruit. That, combined with more strenuous exercise, halved Doug's risk of having a heart attack or dying within five years—and more importantly, it substantially extended the years he will probably spend thriving.

When the cardiac program ended, Doug joined a Y and started running on a treadmill three times a week. At eighty-two, he began lifting weights. "I looked around the gym and saw men and women, whom I knew were as old as I was, walking very vigorously," he said. "I wanted that, too." He built muscle and improved his balance—crucial capacities, given that muscles naturally wither with age, agility lessens, bones grow brittle, and independence can be devastated by a fall. "It started a great wellness loop," Doug said. "More exercise, healthier eating, better sleep, and an improved sense of well-being." At a recent checkup, his doctor said, "Don't change a thing."

The health stage I call Resilience, sometimes called "young" or healthy old age, is a time when you still have the physical capacity to reverse substantial health problems. Most people in the Resilience stage are in their fifties, sixties, and early seventies, but some are exceptionally athletic older people, like Doug von Koss. Length of life is impossible to predict precisely, but people at this stage usually have at least another decade left to live.

This is the time to take inventory, build reserves, and assess what needs shoring up. The major threats to your future well-being will be: physical weakness, isolation, heart disease, lung disease, diabetes, and dementia. You can build bulwarks against them—and prolong your time in Resilience—by exercising, eating better, and widening your circle of friends and passionate interests. Lifestyle habits—especially smoking, being sedentary, eating poorly, and drinking too much alcohol—are responsible for 70 percent of the degenerative diseases that make later life difficult. Change these habits, even after the age of fifty-five, and you can cut your health risks as much as sevenfold—a better payoff than almost all drugs.

I don't mean to suggest that food asceticism and strenuous exercise will ward off death and decline forever. They won't really make you younger next year, though they may keep you happier, stronger, and more functional. Given that our bodies age at the cellular level in more than five thousand specific ways, there's little point in strengthening physical muscles without developing the spiritual and social strength to cope with the inevitable loss of powers, and with death itself. But before you must accept the things you cannot change, you can seize the time to prepare for what's ahead, and to change the things you can.

BUILDING RESERVES

In developed countries, few people die of disease in the first half of life. Most early deaths result from accidents, violence, drug overdoses, and suicide. In late midlife, the picture changes. Cancer becomes a major cause of death in the mid-forties and continues to climb throughout the fifties and sixties. Deaths from heart disease rise in the sixties and seventies, from lung disease in the eighties, and from dementia in the nineties. All cause physical suffering long before they kill, and all are profoundly shaped by how you live.

I suggest you begin by doing what requires the most of you and the least of medicine. The most effective first step (other than quitting smoking) is to walk energetically every day. People over sixty-five who do so increase their lung capacities, get more oxygen to the brain, and expand the size of the hippocampus, a brain organ crucial to memory. As a side benefit, walking around malls, Farmers Markets, and to downtown coffee shops amplifies social connections, another delightful way of improving health, brain function, and happiness. Most of this is not news. But if you've forgotten the deep pleasure and self-confidence that can follow half an hour or more of aerobic exercise, especially in nature or with a friend, consider reacquainting yourself. Even late in the game, getting more active has huge health benefits.

Exercise becomes more challenging as joints grow creaky and minor injuries heal more slowly. Improvise, adapt, and overcome: get moving in any way that makes you break a sweat and gives you joy. Many people find delight in ballroom dancing, biking, or swimming; others find it easier to get started—and to keep going—by scheduling a regular exercise date with a friend. If your feet or knees hurt, consider upgrading shoes or improving your posture or gait with the help of a podiatrist, a physical therapist, or a practitioner of an alternative approach, like Feldenkrais or the Alexander Technique. Stay flexible and be willing to substitute a new activity whenever one falls by the wayside: if you can't run anymore, try water aerobics; if you lose your partner, explore group activities like Greek or country line dancing. No matter what happens, keep going.

The body's capacity to heal, even at this relatively late date, is astounding. Tom Murphy, a former Associated Press journalist who'd once run a marathon, was sixty-two when he was diagnosed with diabetes. He'd been working a stressful and unsatisfying job and, he said, had "fallen into my mom's habit of eating mostly cookies and ice cream, frozen pizzas, Danishes, and lots of bread."

He took a new job and moved from the San Francisco suburbs to rural Mendocino county. By the time he met his new primary care doctor, he weighed 225 pounds and had a trifecta of late-life warning flags: high cholesterol, high blood pressure, and high blood sugar. His alarmed physician recommended he see a cardiologist immediately and start taking a cholesterol-lowering statin, a blood pressure–reducing diuretic, and the blood sugar–lowering drug metformin.

Tom looked at his friends and family, many of whom were already on these drugs, and saw his own future. "I have a friend who went blind from diabetes, another who can't walk, and a third who died of a heart attack," he said. "All could have changed their diets in their fifties, but waited too long. I wasn't going to make the same mistake."

He took blood pressure medication to lower his stroke risk, but asked for a grace period before adding other medications. What followed was, he said, "a very emotional three months. Changing how I lived and ate became more important than work, friends, reading, even my marriage." He jogged a mile and a quarter every morning, starting at a snail's pace and gradually increasing his speed and distance. He stopped eating all foods with added sugar, and other "things that had made my life 'richer.'"

He struggled to change his sleep patterns. He experienced the highs of exercise and the lows of accompanying muscle pain. He wrestled with the drug-like withdrawal effects of quitting sugar, and, as he put it, "the stress of facing multiple life-threatening diseases." To keep going he kept a diary of what he ate and when he exercised, and turned for support to his wife and to a friend who successfully managed her Type 1 diabetes without medication.

Three months later, his cholesterol level was normal for the first time in his life, and so was his blood pressure. His blood sugar levels have fallen more than a third and are now just a hair above normal. His diet is based on fresh vegetables from his wife's garden and smaller amounts of lean turkey, cheese, brown rice, whole wheat bread, and sugar-free jam. Every day he jogs two miles and rides his bike. He weighs 170 pounds and takes no medications. "Yes, it was hard," he said. "It's still hard. But my doctor is very happy and I'm never going back."

FINDING ALLIES IN PREVENTIVE MEDICINE

The most helpful physician at this stage is a good primary care doctor who will coach you to prevent disease. It's not enough to get a yearly lecture on smoking, drinking, or your weight. You want someone who will enthusiastically refer you to physical therapy, or to an effective support group, such as Alcoholics Anonymous, a smoking cessation group, or the diabetes prevention classes offered at many local Ys and covered by Medicare. If your blood pressure, cholesterol, or blood sugar remain high despite lifestyle changes, talk to your doctor about medication: the payoffs are significant for people with a decade or more of life ahead.

The need for a geriatrician—a physician who specializes in the aging body—may not yet seem urgent. But one way or another, it's crucial to find a doctor who cares about you as a whole person long before a health crisis. Many fine doctors who refuse new Medicare patients will continue to treat older people with whom they have established relationships. Look for someone who genuinely cares about his or her patients—and if you're not happy, switch. Now is the time to find someone who will be with you for the long haul.

If your primary care doctor is older than you are, consider finding someone younger who won't retire before you die and has an office close by. (The same goes for dentists, hairdressers, and car mechanics: a twenty-mile drive that is easy today may be harder tomorrow.)

Take advantage of every opportunity to establish rapport with a single doctor who will act as your point person in the world of fragmented medicine that most of us encounter. Ask your doctor to look up from the computer, and to give you a full physical examination. Medicare and some private insurance now reimburse for various "wellness" appointments, including an introductory visit, yearly cognitive assessments, and advance care planning.

Use them to help your doctor get to know you well, and to make sure that you share the same goals.

WEIGHING MEDICAL RISKS

Taking advantage of what he calls Medicare's "bumper-to-bumper warranty," Doug von Koss has had cataract surgery and two knee replacements. They were great moves, postponing further disability, reducing pain, and keeping him happily driving and exercising. But with age, the risks of many procedures rise. "The physiology of the aging body is different: more vulnerable, and more susceptible to the adverse effects of drugs, tests, and operations," cautions Iona Heath, MD, a former president of the Royal College of General Practitioners in the United Kingdom. "This is not ageism; it is person-centered care." Make sure you understand the goal of any proposed treatment: Will it improve how you function day to day, or, in exchange for the hope of more time on earth, are you risking making an existing disability worse? Some people end up with worse pain after back surgery, an outcome common enough to have earned the name "failed back surgery syndrome." Get a second opinion from a physiatrist or other informed non-surgeon, and before agreeing to surgery, try a year of intense physical therapy or a back pain management program.

Just as it's a gamble to buy the first year of a new car model, it is dangerous to be a guinea pig for a medical innovation. Many new medical devices targeted at aging people enter the marketplace with little vetting, thanks to a loophole in Food and Drug Administration (FDA) regulations. Some of these grandfathered-in devices, like metal-on-metal hip implants that crippled patients by shedding metal shavings into their tissues, pose "great safety risks," three eminent doctors warned in the *New England Journal of Medicine.* "Implanted body parts," they noted, "cannot be recalled as easily as defective auto parts."

Above all, guard your brain. It is the keystone of continued independence and freedom. People over sixty are much more vulnerable to "postoperative cognitive impairment" immediately after surgery, and are more likely to still be coping with confusion and memory difficulties three months later. Open-heart surgery requiring hours on a heart-lung pump sometimes fixes a heart valve while wreaking irreversible cognitive damage. You may consider it a poor trade-off to gain extra years of life if you will spend them incarcerated in a locked "memory unit."

GETTING TO KNOW THE NEIGHBORS

Loneliness is a health risk. It's common among older people when their close friends and spouses die, marriages and relationships break up, or grown children move far away. A quarter of Americans now live alone, and married women are quite likely to outlive their mates and experience widowhood. If your love of solitude has deepened into isolation, or you are cocooning within a couple, you might consider making a conscious effort to befriend or mentor younger people, especially neighbors. In a pinch, they may be of more practical help than a family member half a continent away.

My neighbor Paul Reck, an eighty-eight-year-old retired contractor, keeps a plastic container of dog treats by the open door of the garage where he builds scale-model replicas of yachts for boat owners. He's gotten to know all the dogs that pass by on the sidewalk—and their masters. I know I can count on Paul for help putting together an IKEA bookcase or fixing a damaged tea kettle. Paul knows he can count on another neighbor, Barry, for help with his computer problems. Paul's children live hours away. When he or his wife, Nancy, need help, neighbors will step in.

I suggest you consider your own ways to widen and deepen your next-door relationships and to transform them into sources of mutual support. Can you turn neighbors into friends, and friends into honorary siblings? If you're single or widowed, might you rent a bedroom to a foreign student, invite a friend to become a roommate, or enter a pact with a friend to support each other in sickness and in health, the way married couples do?

Don't discount more casual connections, like those formed by babysitting for a younger family down the block, picking something up for a sick friend, or taking in the mail and feeding the dogs when a neighbor goes on vacation. In the future, when you need a prescription picked up or a ride to the doctor, you may feel less shy about asking. Courtesy, neighborliness, and exchanges of favors are pleasant amenities earlier in life. For older people who want to stay in their own homes, they are survival skills.

We live in a society that fetishizes independence—a terrific goal for people in their twenties and thirties. But in later life, *interdependence* is well worth cultivating. Have you mostly been a "taker," an "exchanger," or a "giver"? If you've been a taker, think about becoming an exchanger—one who conscientiously keeps track and returns favors, even if a bit mechanically. If you've been an exchanger, consider giving once in a while without thought of return. If you're exhausted by over-giving, consider cutting back on time spent with takers. You need reciprocal relationships now, not people who drain you.

I've noticed that people who live well in old age, and die well at home, have often found a "tribe" among their fellow quilters, singers, or church group members. When they get sick, the clan shows up to help, spreading the burden of caregiving beyond a single exhausted family member.

Above all, I hope you find ways to connect with others that give your life joy and meaning. The better you understand what makes your life worth living, the more fiercely you can keep it in mind as a guide to medical decision-making when you get closer to the end of life. "Elders worthy of emulation," Doug von Koss once wrote, "know they will soon lose life—and so they generously give it away to those around them." Doug leads a monthly singing group for men. He and some friends regularly perform mystical poems, learned by heart, to benefit local charities. When Doug had knee surgery, a favorite grandson flew out from Colorado and helped for five weeks until he could drive again. Friends a generation younger came over and made dinner. Two members of the all-male singing group he leads—his closest tribe—stand ready to drop everything in an emergency. Because he gives to others, others give to him.

KNOWING YOUR MEDICAL RIGHTS

Contemplating death while embracing life is a difficult balancing act in a culture that until recently didn't want to discuss death at all. Finding the courage and wisdom to break this silence, with your doctors and your family, will shape how death ultimately finds you. In the words of TED talker Judy MacDonald Johnston, who helped care for two older friends dying of dementia and cancer, "Thinking about death is frightening, but planning ahead is practical and leaves more room for peace of mind in our final days."

Not long after his near–heart attack, Doug got together with a dozen older people in the home of a friend. He signed papers giving his son the authority to make his medical decisions if he couldn't make his own and filled out an advance directive, or living will, listing the medical treatments he'd want (and not want) if he were comatose or close to dying.

Most people have already been urged repeatedly to fill out these forms. And 70 percent of us haven't. Perhaps it might help to think of an advance directive as not just a piece of intimidating paperwork, but an act of spiritual maturity.

Nothing is more profound than contemplating your feelings about how you want to be treated when you are dying, or how much suffering and disability you are willing to endure in return for more time on earth. Nothing could be kinder to people who love you than to give them clear guidance for the hardest decisions they may ever have to make. And little could be more empowering than protecting yourself from unwanted medical treatments that now, far too often, dehumanize modern death.

The struggle to control the deathbed has been amplified by modern medical technologies, but it isn't new. Throughout history, doctors have sometimes failed to give adequate pain medication, or continued with painful efforts to ward off death, in direct opposition to the wishes of the dying. The medical historian Michael Stolberg recounts in *A History of Palliative Care* that in 1560, Philipp Melanchthon, a Lutheran minister and a close collaborator of Martin Luther, was close to death. His pulse faded, his hands and feet grew cold, and he drifted in and out of consciousness. His physicians repeatedly tried to revive him, first rubbing his limbs, then trying to sit him up, and then anointing him with stimulants. The sixty-three-year-old Melanchthon protested, "Why do you hinder my gentle peace? Just give me peace until the end, it won't be long now." He died shortly thereafter.

In 1791, the Comte de Mirabeau begged his doctors for the gentlest death possible. "Give me your word that you will not let me suffer any unnecessary pain. I want to enjoy unreservedly the presence of all that is dear to me," he said. A leader in the early stages of the French Revolution, Mirabeau, then in his early fifties, was dying of pericarditis, an inflammation of the sac surrounding the heart. A memoir by one of his doctors shows, wrote Stolberg, "just what torments the doctors allowed their patients to suffer out of fear of prematurely ending their lives, and in this case out of a lack of agreement among themselves"—still a familiar problem.

When Mirabeau's pain grew so severe that he could not speak, he asked for a piece of paper and wrote down the word *dormir* (sleep). He was pleading for opium, but his doctor, P. J. G. Cabani, pretended not to understand. He relented later that night, but a second doctor in attendance said the time had not yet come. Hours later, when the two men reached agreement, it was too late to get the drug compounded and brought to the chateau before Mirabeau died. In agony, he cried out, "I'm being cheated," and added "with a mixture of rage and tenderness . . . Oh, the doctors, the doctors! Were you not my doctor and my friend? Did you not promise me you would spare me the pain of such a death? Do you want me to take with me my regret that I trusted you?" These were his last words and, Cabani wrote, they "rang unceasingly in [my] own ears for a long time to come."

The dying and their families say similar things today, and advance directives are the first line of defense. Many people think they can refuse medical treatment only if they're in a coma or within six months of dying. It's also widely believed that the law and the Hippocratic oath, especially the phrase "do no harm," force doctors to prolong life. Neither is true. The United States Supreme Court has affirmed, and all major medical associations agree, that all competent adults have the legal right to refuse any form of medical treatment, or to ask for its withdrawal, at any time, for any reason. It isn't suicide, assisted suicide, homicide, or euthanasia. It's letting nature take its course, and it's your legal and moral right.

For clarifying these constitutional rights, we can thank the parents of a young woman who worked in a cheese factory in the 1980s. Her name was Nancy Cruzan, and she was twenty-five. On a cold January night in 1983, she was driving home alone from a bar outside Carthage, Missouri, when her car skidded on ice and plunged off the road. She was thrown from her car and landed facedown in a water-filled ditch. Paramedics arrived about fourteen minutes later, pounded on Nancy's chest, shocked her heart until it resumed beating, and forced air into her lungs until they began to rise and fall. But Nancy was too brain-damaged to ever again speak or recognize her family. Incapable of eating or swallowing, her body was kept alive by a feeding tube in a state-funded nursing home. But the "self" that her family recognized as Nancy Cruzan was gone.

Six years later, against opposition from the state of Missouri, her devout Catholic parents petitioned the United States Supreme Court for permission to remove the feeding tube that kept their daughter suspended in what one of her doctors called "a living hell." A deeply divided Supreme Court affirmed that all intellectually competent people have the right to refuse medical treatment. A feeding tube, the high court clarified, is a medical treatment. But Missouri could require "convincing evidence" of Cruzan's wishes. (This, and similar rulings, gave rise to the living will.) In 1990, a Missouri lower court accepted additional testimony and permitted the removal of the feeding tube. A day after Christmas, seven years after her fatal accident, Nancy Cruzan was released from the long, technologically interrupted process of her dying.

The Cruzan decision introduced many laypeople to one of the four pillars of medical ethics, that of patient autonomy: the right to determine and refuse medical treatment. (The other three pillars are treating patients justly; benefiting them; and not harming them.) A doctor who agrees to end an unwanted treatment is not violating the Hippocratic oath. She is honoring your autonomy.

The practical reality, however, is that if you don't have the right paperwork, the default protocol in most emergency rooms will be to do everything possible to ward off death, even when doing so is fruitless and amplifies your suffering. Treatment often does not stop until someone says "enough is enough." The following two documents will help you, or those who speak on your behalf, to do so with confidence.

The Durable Power of Attorney for Health Care appoints a medical advocate or decision maker (technically called a "proxy," "medical power of attorney," "health care agent," or "surrogate") to speak for you if you can't speak for yourself. The ideal person lives nearby, knows what matters to you and is willing to assert it, is willing to drop everything in an emergency, gets along with people, and has a strong backbone. Many people choose a spouse or child, but the best choice isn't always a family member. Because I fear that my husband, Brian, may be emotionally overwhelmed if I am gravely ill, I have chosen a friend whom I've known for thirty years. She keeps a cool head, follows through on her commitments, understands my values, communicates clearly, and has no problem with being assertive.

A Living Will or Advance Directive is the next line of protection. This boilerplate document usually covers only moral and medical dilemmas that arise if you are comatose, close to death, or "unlikely to recover." They rarely cover deactivating internal medical devices like defibrillators, or how to make decisions in case of dementia. You can amend yours however you want to, as it will mainly serve as an informal guide for your medical advocate. If you want stricter, more binding limits placed on medical treatment, you or your advocate should ask your doctor to fill out a do-not-resuscitate order (DNR) and a form called a POLST or a MOLST (Physician or Medical Orders for Life-Sustaining Treatment). These documents are signed by a doctor and are more scrupulously honored than advance directives. They are appropriate for all people in frail health, and are fully discussed in Chapter 5, "The House of Cards."

You can get free advance directives from your health plan, and online from the Conversation Project or Mydirectives.com, which will email copies to anyone you want informed. If you are hesitant, I highly recommend "Five Wishes," available for five dollars from AgingwithDignity.org. Clear and simple, it will help you imagine and describe your vision of a "good death," asking, for example, whether you'd like your body massaged with oil, and what poetry, if any, you'd like read to you. Here are some samples:

My Wish for How Comfortable I Want to Be
(Cross Out Any You Do Not Want:)

- I wish to have warm baths often. I wish to be kept fresh and clean at all times.
- I want my lips and mouth kept moist to stop dryness.
- I wish to have religious readings and well-loved poems read aloud when I am near death.

My Wish for How I Want People to Treat Me
(Cross Out Any You Do Not Want:)

- I wish to have pictures of my loved ones in my room, near my bed.
- I wish to have my hand held and be talked to when possible, even if I don't seem to respond to the voice or touch of others.
- I wish to die at home, if that can be done.

My Wish for What I Want My Loved Ones to Know
(Cross Out Any You Do Not Want:)

- I wish to be forgiven for the times I have hurt my family, friends, and others.
- If there is to be a memorial service for me, I wish for this service to include the following (list music, songs, readings, or other specific requests that you have).

Forms are only symbols of the conversations behind them. More important than paperwork is making sure that your family and closest friends accept the reality of death and commit to following your wishes. When there is no consensus within the family, hospitals often listen to the loudest voice in the room, which often means continuing unwanted treatment. To avoid this, I recommend you talk around the kitchen table with people you love, perhaps every New Year's day, sharing stories of deaths that have frightened or inspired you. It may take some family members years to get comfortable with the reality of your eventual death, so give them time but revisit the subject regularly. Go beyond the dry details covered by advance directives, and talk about your ultimate goal: a "good death," whatever that means to you. Do you want to die at home with your dog on the bed? Do you hope to be conscious enough to give your last words and final blessings, or are you more concerned with pain control, even if it makes you drowsy? Do you want to leave a good emotional legacy, by making sure that loved ones are not traumatized by the circumstances of your death? One single woman I know met at a cafe with the friends who'd agreed to be her health care agents and hashed out the details for over an hour before filling out the forms over muffins and coffee.

Once you complete the forms, don't just leave them in a file at home. At a minimum, send copies to your primary care doctor or health system, to family members, and to anyone you've named to be your advocate. If you simply can't bear to fill them out, I suggest handwriting a letter to whomever will probably make your medical decisions—and mailing it. Tell them what makes your life worth living, and what medical care you'd decline if you could no longer live such a life. Is it crucial to you to love and be loved, to express yourself in words, to garden, to feed yourself, or to sew? What degree of dependence, loss of freedom, pain, or discomfort would be too much to bear? Contemplating your future vulnerability and accepting your mortality shouldn't be minimized as merely checking boxes on a legal form. It is a modern rite of passage.

CARING FOR THE SOUL

Doug is a creature of habit. Every morning he makes his bed, meditates for twenty minutes, and does his own form of affirmative prayer. He reminds himself that he loves himself and his grandchildren unconditionally and lets "God's love, peace, glory, and light" flow through him. He lights a candle and sends prayers to friends whom he knows are sick or close to dying. He makes a mental list of what he's grateful for: that he has a roof over his head, that the wolf is not at the door, that he's got another day to play.

The first two-thirds of life are usually dedicated to learning skills; building a life, a career, and a family; and achieving worldly status. The last third of life has developmental tasks of its own. These generally involve shifting from individualistic striving to greater generosity, and reflecting on what all that work meant. The challenge, and the satisfaction, is to give back to the world something of what you've learned and become. Quiet reflection can aid in the shift from self-absorption to generosity, from striving to letting go, from mourning losses to accepting what is.

Many people return to their childhood religions in later life, or explore other approaches to spirituality. Consider doing so, perhaps by spending half an hour in silence at the same time each day. You might get up before the rest of the household and find a private spot that you can make beautiful with a flower, photo, or view. Some people just sit, enjoying the sensation of breathing, and letting their thoughts come and go. Others say prayers, read poetry or religious texts, or follow a recorded guided meditation. The key is to find a practice that nurtures you, and to do it faithfully, at the same time each day, until your body gets used to the routine. Daily rituals of simply *being* rather than *doing* become more important as time goes by. When death comes, you need to be comfortable with simply being, because there is nothing left to do but let go.

Consider making the contemplation of death a part of your spiritual practice, as do many wisdom traditions. It won't make you die any sooner and it may help you appreciate your life today more keenly. "I am of the nature to grow old," goes a chant repeated each day by monks and nuns in many Buddhist temples:

> There is no way I can escape growing old.
>
> I am of the nature to get sick. There is no way I can escape getting sick.
>
> I am of the nature to die. There is no way I can escape death.
>
> Everything and everyone I love will change. There is no way I can escape being separated from them.
>
> My deeds are my only companions. They are the ground on which I stand.

Around the world in the autumn, during Rosh Hashanah services, Jewish congregations recite that only G-d knows who, in the following year "shall perish by fire and who by water; who by sword, and who by beast; who by hunger and who by thirst." A human being is "as the grass that withers, as the flower that fades, as a fleeting shadow, as a passing cloud, as the wind that blows, as the floating dust, yea, even as a dream that vanishes." I find these natural images beautiful and comforting. They remind me that transience, sickness, aging, and death are not the signs of failure they've come to seem in our can-do society. We are part of an eternal cycle of birth, growth, and decay.

Ways to Prepare:

- Build your physical, social, and spiritual reserves, start planning for a good death, and reverse health problems while you still can.
- Start with what requires the most from you and the least from medicine. Get half an hour or more of vigorous, pleasurable exercise every day.
- Get support from Alcoholics Anonymous, Food Addicts Anonymous, a Diabetes Prevention class at the Y, or a Freedom from Smoking clinic. If your blood pressure, cholesterol, or blood sugar remain high, take medication.
- Find a doctor or a health system that emphasizes prevention, remains accessible if you stop driving, and will be with you for the long haul.
- Get to know neighbors, cultivate friendships with younger people, help friends who are sick, and find ways to mentor and to give.
- Pick a medical advocate (formally known as a medical power of attorney, proxy, health care agent, or surrogate) and talk openly about your fears and wishes.
- Sign an advance directive, free online from The Conversation Project and mydirectives.com, or fill out the "Five Wishes," version, $5 from AgingwithDignity.org, P.O. Box 1661, Tallahassee, FL 32302.
- Prepare not only for death, but for a period of prolonged disability. Fill out forms to allow a trusted friend or spouse to be your "authorized representative" with Medicare, access your medical records, and act as your "durable power of attorney for finances."
- Get your family on the same page. Talk about what a "good death" means to you.
- Create a simple daily spiritual practice, including half an hour of quiet time and a gratitude list, to feed your soul.

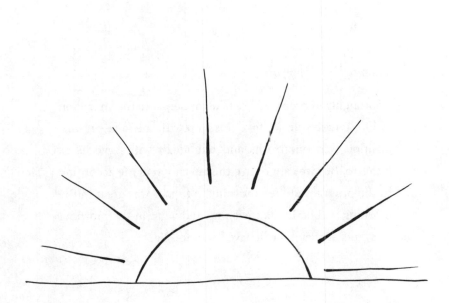

CHAPTER 2

Slowing Down

When Less Is More • Simplifying Daily Life
Finding Allies in Slow Medicine, Geriatrics, and a Good HMO
Reviewing Medications • Reducing Screenings
Making Peace with Loss

Thoroughly Unprepared

Thoroughly unprepared, we take the step into the afternoon of life. Worse still, we take this step with the false presupposition that our truths and our ideals will serve us as hitherto. But we cannot live the afternoon of life according to the program of life's morning, for what was great in the morning will be little at evening and what in the morning was true, at evening will have become a lie.

—CARL JUNG

To do nothing is also a good remedy.

—HIPPOCRATES

You may find this chapter useful if you recognize yourself in some of the following statements.

- It took some effort to blow out all the candles on your last birthday cake.
- You sometimes say "I'm not who I used to be," if only to yourself.
- You see at least two "-ologists": a nephrologist, pulmonologist, urologist, endocrinologist, gastroenterologist, neurologist, or cardiologist.
- You take at least three medications regularly.
- Your physical reserves are thinner. A cold, flu, or minor injury flattens you for a week.
- Your cognitive margins are thinner, too. You sometimes feel confused if you drink too little water, get too little sleep, or pick up a urinary tract infection.
- You're slowing down, and your satisfactions are shifting. You water-walk rather than hike, do t'ai chi rather than salsa, take photographs rather than bike.
- You're not in a nursing home. You don't fall frequently. You can still get out of a chair on your own and walk half a mile under your own power on flat ground. (If any of these are a problem, it is a sign of advanced frailty, and you may want to skip to Chapter 5, "House of Cards.")

WHEN LESS IS MORE

Laura Lamar is a registered nurse, attorney, and hospital risk manager in Chicago. Her father was a pharmaceutical salesman. Years ago, she took a vacation on the central California coast and struck up a conversation in a restaurant with a retired teacher in her late seventies named Marj. The two women quickly bonded: both had wicked senses of humor and plenty of joie de vivre. Marj had come into her own after the death of her husband, an architect, and she was making the most of the time she had left.

The two kept in touch. Whenever Laura was on the West Coast, she and Marj got together for cocktails and outings. Time passed. Marj had a few mini-strokes, turned ninety, sold her house, and moved into an assisted living complex in Monterey with a view of the sea. Her balance grew wobbly. She got dizzy frequently and sometimes lost her train of thought. She started using a walker. But the friendship stayed strong and Laura kept visiting.

One summer day, as the two were sitting down to lunch in the residence dining room, Marj realized she'd forgotten her mealtime medications and asked Laura to go to her unit for them. In the kitchen cabinet, Laura found twenty-two pill bottles neatly lined up, prescribed by six different doctors and filled at four different pharmacies. "Nobody had any oversight," said Laura. "It was a disaster waiting to happen."

Marj was taking drugs for hip pain, sleeplessness, constipation, itchy skin, high blood pressure, acid reflux, and other common late-life miseries. For high blood pressure, her cardiologist had prescribed Lopressor, which can cause insomnia, so another doctor had prescribed a sleeping pill. A second blood pressure medication, Lasix, was making her skin itch, and for that she was taking Benadryl. The Benadryl made her constipated, so she was told to take Dulcolax, a suppository that can cause dizziness. And so it went. Almost every drug on the shelf had a side effect that had led to a new drug that had led to yet another drug to counteract yet another side effect. Dulcolax, Benadryl, and another of her drugs, Tagamet, all caused dizziness, a serious risk for an elderly woman with brittle bones whose balance was unstable enough to require a walker. Benadryl and the sleeping pills are also anticholinergics, an insidious group of commonly prescribed drugs that befuddle thinking and substantially increase the likelihood of developing dementia.

Laura returned to the dining room with a few of Marj's pill bottles in hand and sat down with her friend. "Marj," she said. "This is really, really dangerous. I would have a difficult time managing all these different medications—and you're ninety-two! Do you mind if I have a talk with your son?"

Later that night, she phoned one of Marj's three sons, all of whom lived more than five hours away near the Oregon border. "This is not my business," she said. "But I'm going to put my nose in because I love your mother." She laid out the situation: the pills, the numerous doctors and pharmacies, the right hand not knowing what the left was doing. Laura suggested a "medication review" with a geriatrician—a specialist in the health problems of old age. After a prolonged search—there are only 7,500 geriatric specialists nationwide for an older population of over twelve million—her son found one thirty miles from his mother's home and set up an appointment. Marj put all her medications in a paper bag, got in the car her son hired, and went.

In the geriatrician, Marj finally had a doctor who looked at her as a whole person, rather than a collection of malfunctioning organs. Over the course of the following year, her new "umbrella doctor" weaned her off Benadryl, Lopressor, Dulcolax, and another fourteen of her medications. The process was slow. Her doctor tried drugs with less drastic side effects, reduced dosages gradually, and recommended nondrug alternatives. Marj began swimming five days a week rather than two, which reduced her hip pain. She ate more fiber-rich fruits and vegetables, which diminished her constipation and acid reflux. By the time the year was over, she was taking five prescriptions, saving money, and feeling better. "Her mind was clearer, she wasn't dizzy anymore, her gait and balance were better, she was sleeping better, and she was no longer losing her train of thought," Laura said. "She just needed someone to stand up for her."

Decline, as experienced in the phase I'm calling Slowing Down, is more often felt than seen. Eyes cloud, joints ache, muscles wither, stamina thins, the immune system weakens, bones grow brittle, minor slips of memory bedevil the day. Maladies accumulate.

The medicine cabinet fills with pill bottles, the calendar with doctors' appointments. The body becomes increasingly vulnerable to tiny blows it once shrugged off. Recovery takes longer, and sometimes people never get back to their old "normal." Most people slowing down are in their seventies or older, but some people in their fifties and sixties who are coping with several chronic illnesses are keenly aware they're in this stage.

Continue with the lifestyle changes suggested in the previous chapter, especially exercise, as it will lengthen your time on a high plateau of decent functioning. But one way or another, decline will come. Living the happiest, healthiest possible life is made easier by simplifying daily routines, creating a coordinated team out of a fragmented jumble of doctors, making peace with loss, and understanding the limits of medicine in the face of advanced age and chronic illness.

SIMPLIFYING DAILY LIFE

As energy becomes a precious and limited resource, simplifying is a survival skill. I've learned to beware "the disease of one more thing"—the attempt to squeeze just one more movie, dinner, car trip, or party into a weekend. My husband and I find that when we do less, we enjoy what we *do* do, more. We try to let go of the unimportant and stick with what gives us the most meaning, comfort, and joy. This is a fine time to think about what you hold dear and make sure you are spending your precious life doing it.

Moving to a smaller house, reducing the size of a lawn and the number of mutual fund accounts, putting bills on auto-pay, and decluttering possessions can help you stay independent longer. Keep the tasks of daily life manageable as energy and mental clarity wane. You can also apply the principle of simplification to the doctors you see, the health screenings you permit, and the pills you take.

FINDING ALLIES IN SLOW MEDICINE, GERIATRICS, AND A GOOD HMO

This is a time to reorient your expectations of medicine. What worked when you were younger may not work now. Earlier, the rapid deployment of tests, drugs, and surgeries might have meant the difference between living and dying. But fast medicine can expose aging, fragile bodies to unnecessary risk. Thoughtful, well-coordinated, less aggressive care, supervised by a single doctor, often produces better results. Look for medical allies in geriatrics, primary care, and family medicine, all of whom understand that the health problems of later life are usually caused by multiple factors. What often works best is not a silver bullet, but a lot of modest tinkering.

First formulated by cardiologists in Italy in 2002, the philosophy of Slow Medicine was popularized in the United States by the late Dennis McCullough, MD, a geriatrician at Dartmouth Medical School and author of the landmark 2008 caregivers' manual *My Mother, Your Mother: Embracing "Slow Medicine," the Compassionate Approach to Caring for Your Aging Loved Ones.* Slow Medicine for elders, as McCullough described it, is characterized by medical minimalism, thoughtful collaborative decision-making, and protection from overtreatment. He cautions that at this health stage, "ill-considered testing, drugs, or medical procedures may pose a greater threat than taking no action at all. Poor sleep, indigestion, incontinence, constipation with soiling, and depression are seldom 'fixed' by a drug alone." Look for doctors who take time to create a relationship of trust. Try to find someone who asks about symptoms, takes a careful medical history, touches you, listens, and thinks things through without haste. In the words of cardiologist and Slow Medicine pioneer Alberto Dolara, "To do more is not necessarily to do better."

Given the gaps in our health care system, this may prove impossible. But it's worth a try. Unfortunately, doctors who work as solo practitioners and are paid on a fee-for-service basis are not reimbursed well for giving any patient this kind of thoughtful care. "Spending proper time to deal with several medical issues in one visit," said one former primary care physician, "can take an hour . . . and more time after that for phone calls, notes, and paperwork. Medicare does not pay the $300 to $400 per hour that it takes to run an office, so having such patients is a losing proposition. This is why primary care physicians refer them to specialists and neglect to discuss the big picture." The result is a collection of specialists who don't talk to each other.

For this reason, many good primary care doctors have fled to health maintenance organizations (HMOs) where they are paid on salary and freed from the headaches of running a small office. If you're lucky enough to live in an area with a good HMO or Medicare Advantage plan, and your health problems are not exotic, consider leaving fee-for-service medicine for an HMO.

All-under-one-roof HMOs, like the sprawling, highly rated Kaiser Permanente systems, provide your health care for a set monthly fee or, if you're over sixty-five, via a Medicare Advantage program. Because they are responsible for all your medical costs, HMOs have a vested interest in keeping you healthy and out of the hospital.

Your medical care is usually better coordinated, and HMOs like Kaiser often score high on national ratings of quality and safety. They aren't reimbursed per procedure, so you aren't given treatments because they're remunerative rather than good for you. HMOs often offer classes and support groups to help you to prevent falls or diabetes, thus helping you to stay in charge of your own health. Their doctors make their decisions using "evidence-based medicine"—providing treatments with proven benefits rather than those favored on the basis of a random combination of tradition, physician habit, "gut instinct," reimbursement incentives, and pharmaceutical promotions.

HMOs aren't for everyone. Their doctors also juggle too many patients in too little time. Seeing a specialist requires a referral from your primary care doctor. An HMO doctor won't prescribe a new drug because you saw an ad on television and it won't pay to send you to the nation's expert in your disease unless you can prove it to be "medically necessary" via a time-consuming process.

When you're young and healthy, or have a rare cancer that benefits from specialty treatment, these restrictions may persuade you to keep your options open. In a one-off health crisis, you (or someone who loves you) may have the time and energy to sift through Internet rankings and find a specialist who takes your insurance. But as you age, and your garden-variety health problems multiply, consider the time and energy costs of all that chaotic and fragmented free choice. Many Medicare Advantage programs have lower monthly premiums than traditional fee-for-service Medicare and others offer perks like exercise programs, dental care, and eyeglasses.

If you are lucky enough to live in an area with a Kaiser Permanente organization, or another one of the excellent nonprofit Medicare Advantage plans listed in the back of this book, I strongly suggest checking it out. Advantage plans have a built-in financial incentive to offer better coordinated care to people with multiple health problems, and a better record in caring for the dying. "On almost every quality metric for end-of-life care, terminally ill patients enrolled in Medicare Advantage plans received better care than those enrolled in fee-for-service Medicare," bioethicist Ezekiel Emanuel, a health policy consultant to the Obama administration, wrote in JAMA in 2018. Fewer were hospitalized or admitted to an ICU in their last three months, more enrolled in hospice care, and more died at home rather than in a nursing home.

But the quality of Advantage Plans vary wildly by region. Speech therapist Amy Lustig cautions that many of her clients had access to a better array of covered services when they were in standard Medicare. Check the annual listings of the stellar ones in *US News and World Report*.

In an area without a good freestanding HMO or Medicare Advantage plan, ask around for a regional nonprofit health system with a good local reputation, started by community leaders, with a tradition of collaboration among diverse providers (such as doctors, hospitals, nursing homes, and home care agencies). Then find insurance that covers it.

Another option, if you can afford it, is to join the "concierge practice" of a good primary care doctor. In exchange for a fee (ranging from about $100 a month to many thousands) on top of usual health insurance costs, these doctors devote more time to fewer patients. The phrase may sound snooty, but many concierge doctors are dedicated to delivering time-intensive, high-quality medical care and have patched together a funding model, within a broken system, that permits them to do so. The people I know in concierge practices tend to be much more satisfied with their first-line medical care.

REVIEWING MEDICATIONS

Americans have the dubious distinction of being the most medicated people on earth. With a few notable exceptions, all this pill-taking has not produced significant improvements in health. More than two-fifths of Americans over sixty-five are on more than four medications, and many of those drugs increase their risk of falling, developing dementia, or damaging a vital organ. Medication reactions in people over sixty-five account for a quarter of all emergency room visits and half of all hospitalizations for medication errors, some of which prove fatal. The problem is so widespread that it's earned its own medical label: polypharmacy.

Because your kidneys and liver now work less efficiently, drugs remain longer in your tissues and create more side effects. A medication that causes grogginess may be no worse than a hangover for a young person with the surplus neural connections that scientists call "cognitive reserve." The same side effect might cause an older person to fall or to forget about a pot on the stove, prompting pressure from anxious adult children to make a premature and unnecessary move to an assisted living complex.

The root cause of most overmedication is having multiple doctors write prescriptions. The long-term solution is better coordinated medical care, and the interim solution is to simplify your drug regimen. If you are on more than five medications, set up an appointment for a medication review (and no other purpose) with your primary care doctor, a geriatrician, or a pharmacist with specialized knowledge of geriatrics. (You can also consult the website

Drugs.com, or the *Physician's Desk Reference,* available at most libraries.)

Put all pill bottles, including supplements, in a paper bag. Ask the practitioner about the purpose of each drug, and whether it could be causing a bothersome symptom, especially dizziness, falling, or confusion. Is it amplifying, canceling out, or interacting with another drug on your list? Does it increase your risk of dementia? Is it the lowest effective dose of the cheapest, safest option? Is it working? If you haven't noticed a positive effect after six weeks, can you drop it? Was it prescribed to address another drug's side effect? If so, might you be better off skipping both drugs and just tolerating the original problem?

My watchword here is discernment. Controlling blood pressure and blood sugar, for instance, is proven to save lives and postpone disability. Effective pain management is equally critical, because people in pain exercise less, feel more miserable, get isolated, and function poorly. But I suggest turning a cold eye on the following drugs because of the risks they pose to balance, brain, or continuing independence:

Cholesterol-lowering statins have dubious advantages for people over seventy with no history of heart disease. The benefits, in the form of reduced risk of a heart attack and stroke, are minimal for anyone likely to live less than another decade. Side effects can include fatigue, cognitive impairment, diabetes, and muscle pain and damage, all of which increase fall risk. If you are suffering a difficult side effect, geriatrics specialist Eric Widera, MD, of the University of California medical school in San Francisco, suggests that you and your doctor ponder dropping them.

Drugstore painkillers are useful in moderation, but not harmless. Ibuprofen can raise blood pressure, and repeated overdoses can cause kidney damage severe enough to require dialysis. Many people with chronic pain benefit from low round-the-clock doses of Tylenol (acetaminophen), but overdoses are the nation's leading cause of liver failure. Aspirin in excess can cause stomach bleeding. Rotate minor painkillers and don't take more than labels recommend. Explore managing pain with nondrug remedies, such as yoga, massage, meditation, exercise, physical therapy, or mindfulness-based stress reduction (MBSR), offered by many hospitals and health systems.

Anticholinergics radically increase your risk of developing dementia. They are contained in many over-the-counter and prescription drugs for sleeplessness, allergies, acid reflux, colds, incontinence, irritable bowel, muscle spasms, and anxiety. Staying away from them may be the easiest and most powerful way to protect your brain. As a rule of thumb, beware any drug whose label warns against drowsiness, confusion, or operating heavy machinery.

Be skeptical of drugs containing the anticholinergics chlorpheniramine (in Actifed), diphenhydramine (in Benadryl), and loratadine (in Claritin). One or the other is frequently present in drugs like Excedrin PM, Advil PM, Aleve PM, Nytol, Simply Sleep, Tylenol PM, Chlor-Trimeton, Codeprex, and Advil Allergy and Congestion Relief. A landmark study in Washington State involving more than three thousand people, found that those over sixty-five who used anticholinergics heavily were 50 percent more likely to develop dementia than those who took very few. Many anticholinergics are taken for minor problems; find nondrug remedies, or wait it out.

Prednisone and other steroids reduce pain and inflammation by dampening the immune system. They increase the risk of falls and cognitive impairment. Find alternatives unless life is at risk, and even then take the lowest dose for the shortest possible time. Noted side effects include depression, confusion, mood swings, muscle weakening, temporary psychosis, and long-term heart damage.

Benzodiazepines and *sleeping pills* increase dizziness, fatigue, and falls. If you are anxious or suffer from sleeplessness, be cautious about Valium, Librium, Xanax, Ativan, and Halcion. Daniel Hoefer, MD, who oversees serious illness management programs for the Sharp Rees-Stealy Health System in San Diego, suggests aggressively exploring nondrug remedies. Once again, start with what requires the most from you and the least from medicine, before escalating step-by-step to drugs with greater potential for harm. Benzodiazepines are addictive and should be used only short term; weaning yourself must be done very slowly, under a doctor's supervision.

See if incremental fixes will improve your sleep quality, which naturally declines with age. Many people do better when they skip caffeine after noon; get more exercise in daylight; keep a regular bedtime; replace a lumpy mattress; wear socks to bed; shut down computer and TV screens after dinner; and keep the bedroom cool, quiet, and dark, using earplugs and a sleep mask if necessary. Others improve their sleep with bedtime rituals, like drinking chamomile tea; taking a twenty-minute hot bath shortly before bed; making a to-do list for the next day; or listening to a relaxation or self-hypnosis audio. Some people swear by the hormone melatonin, available over-the-counter, but its long-term effects have not been studied.

In all things, don't let the cure be worse than the disease. A leaky bladder, for example, is an embarrassing and common old-age inconvenience—but the Ditropan (oxybutynin) often prescribed is an anticholinergic. When people on it seem befuddled, the antidementia drug Aricept is added, often worsening the original incontinence. Another common side effect of Aricept is a slowed heartbeat, which can lead to the unnecessary implantation of a pacemaker. Better to eliminate both drugs and see whether you are any worse off. Once again, start by exploring nondrug remedies: ask your doctor for a referral to a continence training class, learn to do Kegel exercises, use pads and time bathroom breaks, or try taking a postnatal yoga class to strengthen your internal musculature.

REDUCING SCREENINGS

A "screening" is a search for a health problem in the absence of symptoms. Some, such as Pap tests, have proven their worth by catching treatable diseases early. But they've also led to medical overkill, and geriatrics specialists recommend against many of them because they promote unneeded worry and overtreatment.

The American Academy of Family Physicians, for instance, recommends against a PSA (prostate cancer) test for men over seventy-five without a family history of fast-moving prostate cancer. A high PSA reading often creates emotional pressure to undergo surgery and radiation, which can leave you with incontinence and impotence without extending or improving your life. Most prostate cancers are so slow-growing that older men die *with* them rather than *of* them.

Colonoscopies save lives by detecting precancerous polyps. The United States Preventative Task Force does not recommend them for people over age seventy-five without a family history of colon cancer. They usually require sedation and large co-pays, and they carry a small risk of perforating the colon—a potentially devastating physical setback to an older person. (They are, however, very well reimbursed.) The polyps can take five to ten years to develop into cancerous lesions. If you're unlikely to live that long, or are too fragile to withstand surgery in any case, skip the screening. An annual twenty-dollar noninvasive FIT screening (fecal immunochemical test), or the higher-priced Cologuard, will look for hidden traces of blood in your stool, and will do almost as good a job of detecting problems in your lower colon at a fraction of the cost and risk. You collect a sample in the privacy of a bathroom, put it in an antiseptic bottle, and mail or deliver it to a lab. You can find other "not recommended" screenings, vetted by the relevant medical specialty, on the Choosing Wisely site of the American Board of Internal Medicine (ABIM).

MAKING PEACE WITH LOSS

Loss is a given in this life stage. Grieving—for people who have died, for a job you once enjoyed, for physical powers that are fading—is not depression. Don't pathologize sorrow, it's a healthy and common human emotion. Antidepressants cannot cure it, and many that work well in midlife, such as Prozac, increase the risk of falling.

After his wife, Clydene, died of pancreatic cancer in 2006 at the age of sixty-nine, Doug von Koss spent months mourning her. Clydene had been a knitter and an award-winning quilter, making all her own clothes on her prized Bernina sewing machine. Every closet and drawer, every square inch of their shared house, was stuffed with boxes filled with materials for her crafts.

"Evidence of her passions was everywhere," Doug told me. "A closet bursting with costumes and dresses she had designed and crafted, each with a particular memory for me. The smell of her perfume—Shalimar. Enough fabrics in the basement to supply a quilting society for a year, and enough yarn to make sweaters for two kindergarten classes. There were carefully labeled boxes dedicated to holidays and birthdays, each carrying a memory of friends and family and, of course, Clydene. There was an enormous hole in our home and in my heart."

After the memorial service, he created an altar to Clydene on top of the grand piano in their dining room. Atop a piece of brocade fabric, he placed emblems of his dead wife: her lace handkerchief, a pair of her earrings, a pincushion, her knitting needles, embroidery scissors, a tape measure, a favorite teacup and saucer, and a framed photo of her when she was still radiantly healthy. He covered the altar with a piece of lace, so that most of the time he could see only the vague outline of her precious things.

Each morning, in a private rite marking his transition from husband to widower, he would uncover the altar and have a conversation with Clydene—"sometimes internal, sometimes aloud," he told me. He wept in seemingly endless sorrow. "Sometimes it was really raw, but grief isn't pretty. When I felt complete, I covered the altar and got on with the day."

Occasionally he came across an object or a photo that carried a new memory and placed it on the altar, so that it wasn't static. After months of mourning, he reread the marriage vows they'd taken and came to the place that reads " 'til Death do us part."

He had kept his vows and completed them. Death *had* parted them. He was husband no more. "The sense of loss diminished and a gratitude for what we had took its place," he said. "This was a welcome surprise." He took down the altar and left the company of mourners. He emptied the closets, distributing Clydene's treasures to her friends, her daughter, her daughter-in-law, and her granddaughters. He gave clothes to Goodwill and fabrics to quilters.

One day he felt the urge to paint what had been their bedroom (and was now only his) a burnt orange, even though he was sure she'd have disapproved. Next he painted the bathroom a sea green—surely too bright for her taste. The dining room and living room followed, painted a beautiful Mexican yellow gold. He bought wall-to-wall carpeting, put down new linoleum in the kitchen, and hung up pictures he knew she wouldn't have liked. The colors are unusual, harmonious, and beautiful.

"Her voice was over my shoulder a lot," he said. "*Oh Doug, you're not going to do that, are you?*

"And of course, I did. And clearly, I love it! Rugs, bedding, towels, curtains, upholstery, and much more were changed to accommodate a widower who needed a sanctuary for the long haul," he said. "It is quite enough to carry the memories of our lives together in my heart and imagination. I can visit them at my choosing now, instead of living in a constant reminder of what once was and is no more."

Ways to Prepare:

- Simplify your life, manage your energy, and do what really matters to you.
- Enroll in an HMO or Medicare Advantage plan that provides well-coordinated medical care if there is a good one in your area, or find a geriatrician.
- Schedule a medication review with a doctor or pharmacist once a year, and whenever a new medication is added.
- Above all, guard your brain. Stay away from anticholinergics, which increase your risk of dementia. Be equally cautious about drugs that increase fall risk. For a full list of drugs dangerous to older people, consult the updated "Beers List" from the American Geriatrics Society.
- Question and eliminate unnecessary health screenings by checking the Choosing Wisely website.
- Improvise rites of passage to make peace with loss.

CHAPTER 3

Adaptation

A Moment of Truth • Mapping the Future and Making Plans
Finding Allies in Occupational and Physical Therapy
Disaster-Proofing Daily Life • Making a Move
Practicing Interdependence • Being an Example

Now a Pinion, Next a Spring

I learned with great regret the serious illness mentioned in your letter [and hope] you are entirely restored. But our machines have now been running for 70 or 80 years, and we must expect that, worn as they are, here a pivot, there a wheel, now a pinion, next a spring, will be giving way: and however, we may tinker them up for a while, all will at length surcease motion. Our watches, with works of brass and steel, wear out within that period.

—THOMAS JEFFERSON to JOHN ADAMS, Monticello, July 5, 1814

You may find this chapter helpful if you recognize yourself in some of these statements.

- You know you're not going to "get better." This is the new normal.
- You say "I don't know who I am anymore," if only to yourself.
- You've given up driving.
- People you've helped in the past are helping you now.
- You use hearing aids, a cane, a walker, a Seeing Eye dog, or a wheelchair.
- You need help with some chores of modern life, such as yard work and housework, shopping for groceries, doing your taxes, taking medications on time, cooking dinner, or making phone calls.
- Your health conditions aren't annoyances anymore. They've changed how you live.
- You sometimes worry that you're exhausting your family members.
- You're considering moving into assisted living or in with a relative, or getting more help at home.
- You no longer call the shots around your house, and you know it.

A MOMENT OF TRUTH

It was an early evening in late autumn in Marin County, just across the Golden Gate Bridge from San Francisco. Twilight had fallen. Bronni Galin, an eighty-two-year-old practicing psychotherapist, was driving from her office to her home in the leafy suburb of Mill Valley.

For more than a year, she'd been losing her central vision to age-related macular degeneration. After a couple of fender-benders, she'd promised her two daughters that she'd drive only in daylight. But Daylight Savings Time had just ended, sunset had arrived sooner than she expected, and there she was, driving home at dusk. She was only a couple of miles from the small wooden house in the hills where she'd planned to live until the end of her life.

She felt a soft bump against the right side of her car. She thought she'd hit an animal. She stopped, got out, and tried to find it. She couldn't. Shaken, she drove the rest of the way home at a crawl.

That night she called both daughters, one of whom lived fifty miles to the north and the other in rural New Mexico. It was time, they said, to stop driving. If Bronni had lived in another, more walkable time or place—a Greek island village, perhaps, or a large home shared with extended family, or even the apartment in Brooklyn where she'd grown up—this ultimatum would not have been so devastating.

But suburbs are cruel and poorly designed places for single people of modest means growing increasingly disabled with age. Her house was just beyond walking distance from her office, the grocery store, and the community pool where she water-walked three times a week. There was no local bus service to speak of. Stopping driving, she knew, would drastically reconfigure her life.

Bronni was long divorced. In addition to losing her sight, she was coping with diabetes and painfully arthritic feet. She wore two hearing aids and, even with their help, had increasing trouble

using the phone. She took comfort from her long-term meditation group, where almost everyone was older and struggling with
health problems. "Our bodies," she told me simply, "are failing us."

She knew that if she couldn't get to her office she would have to
retire. If she didn't get to the pool, she might grow weaker, more
disabled, and depressed. If she couldn't shop for groceries . . . well,
that was obvious. The daughter who lived in New Mexico invited
Bronni to move there. But the idea of giving up her home, her
calling, her neighborhood, her meditation group, and her friends
didn't fill Bronni with joy.

She put her home on the market, gave her car keys to the
daughter who lived closest, gave the dining room table to her
other daughter, and put a lifetime of possessions in storage. She
planned to use the money to rent a one-bedroom apartment in
The Redwoods, a retirement community near the center of town.
The Redwoods had van service, social workers, a dining hall, and a
garden with raised beds. It was close to a park and across the street
from a supermarket. When Bronni needed more help, she could
"graduate" to one of its assisted living units or to full-on nursing
care. But the apartment was miniscule, and the rent alone would
be more than $40,000 a year.

Bronni's house sold in a week. At the eleventh hour, she decided against The Redwoods and instead accepted an invitation to
share a two-bedroom apartment, on a ridge in the next town, with
a woman from her meditation group. Her new living situation was
rich in social networks. Her housemate, Julie, was eighty-five, in
good health, and still drove a car. Julie's two grown children lived
nearby; her son was a contractor who helped out with minor
home repairs. Bronni's share of the rent was a third of the cost of
the retirement home. She opted for preserving more autonomy,
patching together an informal support network, and using the
money she saved to hire help when she needed it.

———

She reconfigured her life not by magically becoming less disabled, but by enriching her connections and expanding her sense of "family." A crucial piece of the puzzle was joining Marin Villages, part of a national alliance of older people determined to age in place in their own homes. Modeled on the pioneering Beacon Hill Village, founded in Boston in 2001, Marin Villages is one of more than a hundred similar groups. This rapidly growing movement aims to make neighborhoods more livable for late old age by building networks of mutual support and providing referrals to volunteers and paid professionals like carpenters, home health aides, and housekeepers.

Once she paid her dues of $365 a year, volunteers from Marin Villages gave Bronni rides to the pool, her office, and the grocery store. Someone came over and changed overhead lightbulbs that neither she nor her housemate could safely reach. Another volunteer helped her install new software on her laptop.

Her life is an assemblage of makeshift solutions and compromises. She depends on hired hands and the kindness of friends and strangers. When she can't get a ride from a volunteer, she pays for a taxi, a community paratransit van, or Uber, which she calls by phoning an intermediary agency called "GoGo Grandparent." (She has a flip-phone and can't hail Uber on her own.)

Yes, these are imperfect and impermanent arrangements. Many solutions in this health stage are. But her patchwork of help has transformed what could have been a crippling, autonomy-destroying disability into a major inconvenience. Bronni is still working, cooking her own meals, and doing her water-walking. A downward spiral of isolation, passivity, and inactivity—the likely course had she become homebound in her old house—has been delayed.

Adaptation has had its price. Selling her cherished home, with its lifetime of memories and its magnificent view, was wrenching. Its new owners plan to demolish it and replace it with something grander. One day not long after signing the escrow papers, Bronni got a ride to her old house, looked in the windows, and cried—saying a private goodbye to a beloved place is now a common rite of passage. "I miss my house desperately," she said. "I talk to it. I had the stuff of a lifetime there—the rocks and stones, the old posters."

"My housemate is kind. But now I'm in *her* apartment. It's very different from being in my own space." Maintaining her serenity requires managing lowered expectations, accepting the imperfect, giving herself permission to grieve, and letting go of what once was and is no more. By necessity, she is learning to practice a virtue that the old ascetic and stoic religions called "renunciation": releasing worldly things, or at least accepting that they go away by themselves.

All this has forced Bronni to rethink the basis of her self-respect. "I was the one that helped, not the one that asked," she said. "I had to give up hating to ask for help." Every morning she lies in bed and reckons with the distance between what she used to do and what she can do now. "I need to do everything more slowly," she said. "I always prioritize the most important thing to do that day. I'm not guided by 'shoulds' but what I know is the truth. I tell the truth, no matter how inconvenient, no matter how opposed to the image I'd like to project. I try to be generous and kind with myself. And some priorities never get done."

Disability sometimes arrives suddenly in the form of a stroke, and more often comes on little cat feet, as an accumulation of small impairments. Continuing to shape a good life rests largely on adapting to change, abandoning shame, and accepting help.

Consider reducing your faith in drugs, surgery, and specialists, and increasing your faith in human community and plain common sense.

The right kind of medical care can help. The focus turns away from chasing diagnoses with top specialists and toward modest, practical, so-called ancillary health care workers—social workers, physical therapists, and occupational therapists. All can significantly improve your function and quality of daily life. They are less likely to ask "what's the matter *with* you?" and more likely to ask "what matters *to* you?" Their goal is not to have you running marathons. It's to keep you doing things that give your life joy. It's to slow impairment and to find substitutes for activities you can no longer do in old ways.

You're also likely to need practical support from others: a family member; a handyman; a Meals on Wheels volunteer; and paid assistance. Adjusting isn't easy in a culture that worships an extreme, impractical ideal of independence. One of the spiritual tasks of this health stage is to dismantle this one-sided belief.

Human beings are herd animals. We give and receive help throughout our lives. You may find, to your surprise, that some of those who help you regard it as an honor, a calling, or a chance to deepen intimacy. You may find yourself forced to cultivate old-fashioned virtues, like humility, graciousness, persistence, and flexibility. Older people who've learned to treat other people decently, no matter what their social status, will have an easier time navigating this drastic psychic reorganization. Masters of the Universe who've relied on money or prestige to bend others to their will are likely to have a harder time. Unless you're very rich, the more you can plan for, ask for, and accept help graciously, the happier—and ironically, the more functionally independent—you are going to be.

MAPPING THE FUTURE AND MAKING PLANS

The unfortunate thing about the life stage of Adaptation is that the "new normal" is likely to keep shifting, usually in the direction of further loss of physical and mental powers. Hoping for the best is fine, but if deepening disability is in your future, this is the time to plan—financially, practically, and medically—for the worst. One of the most useful things your doctor can do is to give you a clear sense of your overall health trajectory. If your eyesight is failing, knowing how rapidly blindness is advancing, and how bad it's likely to get, can help you decide when to go for rehabilitation training. (Almost all forms of rehabilitation are more effective when undertaken while you still retain some function.) If you have memory loss, knowing how fast it is moving might motivate you to update your estate plan, to sign new health directives limiting life-prolonging medical care, or to start researching assisted living or a nursing home. Some people, to their surprise, find life in disability sweeter than they expected. Others have the opposite response.

Armed with a clearer vision of the future, you can make practical changes in a timely manner, rather than waiting for a crisis to force change upon you. Kelcy Allwein, a Defense Department analyst who's now sixty-six, developed a rare form of glaucoma in 2013 and underwent surgery. Given that she's single and is likely to be blind for some years before she dies, she matter-of-factly anticipates a series of downsizings, first from her three-bedroom house to an apartment, and from there to assisted living and eventually to hospice care. This practical letting-go has become a private rite of passage. Over the past five years, using a spreadsheet, she's sent her costume jewelry to a charity thrift shop and gotten rid of duplicate dishes and furniture that no longer suit her taste. A library of more than seven hundred religious and inspirational books went to a military chaplain to use or give to others.

She had collected a myriad of china coffee cups as mementos of her travels. Before she let them go, she took photographs and made an album. "Because I've let go of things, I have space to form new memories now," she said. "I am also thinking about putting together audio stories of who I was and who I am becoming in case my eyes get worse. I don't look at it as a kind of death, but as rebirth and renewal—a shedding of old skin for something new.

This is also the time to take a look at your financial plans, especially if your resources are limited. More than a third of baby boomers have less than $50,000 saved for retirement. Forty percent will eventually need practical help for two to five years. Given that residential assisted living can easily cost $100,000 a year, people with less than half a million dollars in savings or home equity, and without long-term care insurance, should organize their finances with an eye to accessing public benefits like Medicaid. Do this at least five years before you think you'll need help.

Medicaid pays for nursing homes for people who've exhausted most of their assets, and provides home health aides and some excellent community support programs. To qualify, you must have a limited income and $2,000 or less in savings, though you may own a house and a car. When you apply, Medicaid will look back at five years of your financial records to prevent you from hiding or transferring assets to appear poorer than you are.

Prepaying for a cemetery plot, or substantially upgrading your house to adapt it to your disability, or paying an adult child or other relative the going rate to help care for you, are all legitimate transfers in the eyes of Medicaid. But buying your son a Jaguar as a gift is not, nor is giving your daughter an early share of an expected inheritance. If you're married, almost all of your spouse's assets must be "spent down" before Medicaid will qualify you, even if you have a prenuptial agreement to keep your finances separate.

The rules are tricky, and you run a serious risk of leaving your surviving spouse with little money for his or her most vulnerable years. If you think you or your spouse may need Medicaid someday, I recommend reading *How to Protect Your Family's Assets from Devastating Nursing Home Costs: Medicaid Secrets* by elder law attorney K. Gabriel Heiser now. It won't answer all your questions, but it does address such arcane matters as how to structure an annuity to avoid impoverishing the surviving spouse. Because rules vary by state, you should also consult a local lawyer specializing in "elder law," with specific expertise in Medicaid.

FINDING ALLIES IN OCCUPATIONAL AND PHYSICAL THERAPY

In Adaptation, you may find your life hopes shifting. Many people and their families now choose to concentrate less on lengthening life, and more on quality-of-life goals, such as delaying physical and cognitive decline; staying out of a nursing home; and creating a life of renewed pleasures, however limited.

The longer you stay active and well socialized, the happier, healthier, and more functional you will be. Ask for referrals to physical, speech, or occupational therapy at every opportunity. Keep doing at least a half an hour of something physical, and hopefully enjoyable, every day, even if it's just trundling to the end of the driveway with a walker or doing stretch-band exercises in a chair.

Perhaps the most important goal is maintaining your ability to get in and out of a chair. (People who can't usually end up in nursing homes.) Seek regular physical therapy to help you preserve this crucial capacity. Medicare once cut off payments for PT when you stopped showing improvement, but a court settlement now requires it to cover as much as you need to maintain your current level of functioning. (Medicare will, however, require additional paperwork to cover more than twenty sessions per year.) If you must pay out of pocket, do so if you can afford it. Or try following along with an exercise class on TV, a video, or Jane Fonda's gentle exercise routines for older people, available on YouTube. One resourceful woman I know brought herself back from a debilitating illness (at the age of 104) by doing Royal Canadian Air Force exercises in bed.

If and when you give up one activity, substitute another. Lois Lieberman, a retired mapmaker for the city of Los Angeles, now ninety-five, ran her first marathon at the age of sixty-nine. After she injured her knee in her early seventies, she shifted to Jazzercise, Pilates, and t'ai chi. "You just have to keep going," she said. "Small fears, you've got to fight them. It's okay to feel sorry for yourself for a short period of time. Then give yourself a hug and go for it. It can be done."

After cataract surgery, she lost her sense of balance. For the first few months, she couldn't even walk with a cane. "I stopped moving," she said. "And then other things started to go." She now exercises on a stair stepper inside her home while holding on to the backs of chairs placed on either side. So far, she's recovered her ability to walk with a cane and hopes for more. "I hope I'm slowly getting back," she said. "In the meantime, I've had a good run."

DISASTER-PROOFING DAILY LIFE

One of the cheapest, easiest, most effective ways to preserve your independence is to reduce your risk of falling. A sailor in a small boat knows that a carelessly coiled line can lead to an entangled foot, a ripped sail, or being thrown overboard. The bumpy seas of late old age also require meticulous hazard reduction. Respect your increased fragility and eliminate every seemingly trivial element that increases your risk. Start with the interior of your own body. If you've been tottering, falling, or nearly falling, shore up your balance and stability. Many people improve their lower-body strength, ankle flexibility, and balance with practices like Pilates, yoga, or t'ai chi. People over the age of seventy who do t'ai chi are half as likely to fall as others their age, and when they do fall, they're half as likely to break a bone. Teachers of this flowing martial art now have studios across the country. An effective alternative, offered by many community groups and health systems, are "fall prevention" classes. Take one.

Aging bodies regulate temperature poorly, and dehydration and overheating can cause dizziness and lead to falling. During heat waves, drink lots of water, go to an air-conditioned movie or tie a wet bandanna around your neck—it's an astonishingly effective form of personal air-conditioning. If you don't see well and need cataract surgery, get it—dim eyesight is a fall risk.

Now check your body's immediate exterior. Give up progressive lenses, as they make it hard to judge uneven ground. Shoes with unstable heels and slippery or flapping soles are no longer inconveniences; they're hazards, so get them fixed. (And throw out high heels if you haven't already.) Finally, look at your home and its surroundings. Ask your primary care doctor to write a referral for an occupational therapist to assess your house for fall hazards and recommend ways to fix them.

An occupational therapist is likely to recommend that you fix tipped pavers on pathways and install handrails on your porch stairs. Add motion-sensors and brighter lights to the driveway, walkway, and decks. Clear flowerpots from outer stairways. Make first and last steps easier to see, with a contrasting color of paint.

Inside the house, an OT will also suggest you get rid of slippery throw rugs or anchor them with a nonslip pad or rug tape. Add grab bars wherever you can. Install brighter lights to interior stairways and halls, with additional switches or motion sensors. Remove clutter from floors, keeping a sharp eye out for magazines, extension cords, and cardboard boxes that are easy to trip over. If you have fallen when rushing to the bathroom at night, add a commode by the bed.

If you are determined to age in place and stay in your own home until you die, imagine deeper disability and plan for it. Take a test drive with a roll-aboard suitcase, from the curbside all the way to your bedroom, to uncover barriers to a wheelchair or walker. Widen doorways to thirty-five inches and remove thresholds.

If you have the money, consider more extensive home improvements, such as bidets, walk-in showers, pull-out drawers in the kitchen, electrical outlets that don't require bending, levers rather than doorknobs for arthritic hands, and brighter LED lighting in laundry rooms and closets so your dimmed eyes can see stains on your clothes. (As I mentioned earlier, Medicaid will not count these expenditures against you, and once you enter the program, you won't have the money.) Renovating a downstairs bedroom and bathroom might help you to live entirely on the ground level when you have to (and only then—going up and down stairs, for as long as you can, will keep you stronger and more functional).

An occupational therapist can also help if some activities, such as dressing on your own, have become difficult. Let go of vanity and follow their recommendations for easy-off clothing and shoes, toilet-seat raisers, tip-proof cups, and slip-proof bowls and place mats. If your range of movement is limited, a long-handled comb can let you brush your own hair, and a "grabber" can reach shelves. Video monitors enlarge book print. Hearing aids make it easier to enjoy your friends and to stay socially engaged. They're a double win: they reduce your risk of further hearing loss, and of dementia.

Many people who've developed disabilities, unfortunately, deny themselves many former pleasures because they are too embarrassed to be seen at the opera using a walker, or attending a dinner party using hearing aids. This is understandable, given our society's shame about aging and disability, which are normal stages of later life. (Many younger people, as Ashton Applewhite puts it in *This Chair Rocks*, are "prejudiced against their future selves.") Get over your embarrassment and internalized shame. Becoming adept with aids will enlarge your independence and your pleasures, and improve your quality of life.

MAKING A MOVE

When Doug von Koss's San Francisco landlord died, he had to leave the rent-controlled house that had been his home for thirty years. He found a smaller rental cottage in a flatter, more walkable neighborhood on the edge of Sebastapol, a bustling market town surrounded by vineyards and apple orchards, fifty miles to the north. A son lives one town away, several close friends a decade younger than him live nearby, and he's now much closer to stores and coffee shops, which is likely to keep him socially connected and physically active if he has to give up driving someday. If you are planning a move, look for a neighborhood friendly to nondrivers, perhaps one with good public transportation or houses or apartments closely packed together. You want to be within walking distance of a supermarket, health club, or coffee shop where you can become a "regular." You might choose an area, or even an apartment building, where a relative or friend already lives. If the region is served by a good nonprofit health plan or high-quality HMO, so much the better.

Consider seeking out a neighborhood that already has a "Villages" mutual aid network, or a place where you might help start one. If you can afford it, explore getting a place with an extra bedroom served by its own private bathroom, kitchenette, or entrance. All are great attractions for a future paid caregiver, a younger student lodger, or a roommate.

If you are choosing a retirement community, I suggest you visit at least three and ask yourself the following questions:

- Can you walk to interesting places, or do you have to be driven everywhere by van?
- Can you "test drive" by staying a week before making a commitment that may be difficult to reverse? This is not a choice to make in a panic.
- Can you "graduate" to skilled nursing onsite and get more help when you become too fragile for independent or assisted living? Moving can be difficult during a major health crisis.
- What is the policy regarding minor falls? Will they send you to the emergency room whether or not you want to go? Can you negotiate an exception?
- Is it served by a physician or nurse house call service?
- What is the philosophy regarding the end of life? Does the staff make an effort to honor do-not-resuscitate orders and other medical directives, and make sure they travel with you to the hospital? Are staff comfortable with palliative care, hospice, and "comfort care"?
- How does the place feel on a gut level? Some fancy places with great interior decor turn out to be bureaucratic, profit-oriented, and devoid of warmth. Some modest family-run "board and care" homes, housing a handful of older people, provide a great deal of comfort and love.
- Will you find friends with similar interests? The Redwoods, in my liberal town, is full of artists and activists. My friend Anne's parents, a retired general and his wife, chose a retirement home outside Washington, D.C., exclusively populated by former military people.
- Does the place have a mission other than profit? Many well-regarded places were founded by religious groups. The excellent Kendal Homes were started by Quakers. Little Sisters of the Poor and Nazareth Homes were founded by

Catholic nuns, and many retain a tender, caring feeling. The Beatitudes Campus in Phoenix, Arizona, founded by the local protestant Church of the Beatitudes, is a national leader in flexible, imaginative, noncoercive care for people with Alzheimer's disease. Jewish Homes for the Aged are often outstanding. Masonic Homes, and others run by community nonprofits, will often let you stay on if you run out of money, helping you access charitable grants or Medicaid. All are open to people of all religions.

PRACTICING INTERDEPENDENCE

When disability strikes, many families are stunned to discover that Medicare pays for little to no home health aides or nursing home care, beyond rehab for a limited time after a three-day hospital admission. Unless you qualify for Medicaid, most of your help will come from volunteers, family, and friends, supplemented by a patchwork of limited services provided by local nonprofit agencies and businesses.

This rip in the national safety net creates a strong incentive for staying as functional as you can, for hiring small amounts of help sooner rather than later, and for learning to graciously receive from people who are fond of you. It's often wiser to pay for some services, or to accept small bits of assistance from many friends, than to tough it out until you or a single caregiver collapses.

Now is the time to draw on the social "bank account" you created in the Resilience phase, when you mentored younger people and helped out your neighbors. The wider your network of support, the better. If someone says "Let me know how I can help," give them one small, manageable, repeating task, like doing the laundry every Monday, or taking you out to lunch once a month. It's better to have a dozen people pitch in a little than insist on the exclusive help of one exhausted spouse. If, when you were stronger, you did favors for others, you may now feel more comfortable asking others to do the same for you.

Caregiving is a two-way street. Encourage your caregivers to practice compassion for themselves as well as for you. If you can afford some paid home care, give family caregivers a daily break and one day "off" per week. Or consider reducing their burdens by outsourcing some of *their* routine tasks. You might hire a high school student to do *their* grocery shopping, or drop off their dry cleaning, or drive you to your medical appointments.

Caregiving can be one of the most exhausting and lonely roles that most of us will ever experience (and most of us, especially women, will fill it repeatedly) given that families are scattered across the country, government support is minimal, and social networks are often frayed. Caregivers experience significantly less stress when they feel they are helping effectively, and that you appreciate it. Every time someone's presence in your life gives you joy, or the help provided allows you to keep doing something you love, say so out loud. The daily practice of gratitude, which you may have begun earlier, can have real payoffs now.

If one family member is shouldering most of the burden, consider paying him or her an hourly wage at the going rate, and letting other family members know about it. This can reduce future bitterness and is fairer to the one who puts in years of personal and financial sacrifice only to receive the same share of inheritance as those who did little but kibitz from afar. As mentioned earlier, such family payments will not delay your admission to Medicaid, as long as the pay is reasonable and your record-keeping is good.

Explore resources in the wider community as well. If your town offers a good day program for older people, consider it. These programs give older people opportunities to make art, play mah jongg, sing, go on outings to movies and museums when they can no longer drive themselves, and eat lunch together. They reduce boredom and isolation, improve mood and health, and give care-givers a lifesaving respite. Enrolling someone you love, or going yourself, can feel like a blow to your dignity, I know. Even when my mother was nearly broken from nonstop caregiving, our family felt too humiliated to consign my increasingly demented father to the company of others like him. But we were defending the pride of the man he used to be, not the man he had become.

So my poor father sat for years alone in the living room at home, dignified, bored, and lonely. He was a prisoner of our shame. He loved to paint and to write and enjoyed the company of other people. A day program could have given him those things in his radically changed circumstances. Explore what's offered in your area, and don't follow our bad example.

If you're in a financial position to hire home help, you may be in for an unexpected boon: a surprisingly tender and close near-family relationship. Some home health aides look on their profession as a calling, and are gifted at it. The bonds they develop can be of as-tonishing intimacy. Honor them, if you can, by paying above mini-mum wage and contributing to their Social Security accounts, if they have them. (Many, however, prefer to be paid under the table.)

If you're comfortable with interviewing, hiring, and firing people, you may do well finding your own in-home caregivers via Craigslist or word of mouth. Home care agencies keep more than half of the hourly fee, and usually require a four-hour minimum shift. My family hired caregivers privately, because we wanted more flexible shifts. We found skillful, kind, remarkable people by paying them nearly double the going rate—and no more than we would have paid an agency. Think about what will work best for *you*. Don't settle. You may cycle through several not-so-good caregivers before you find the extraordinary ones with whom you click.

This is a complex relationship, and I recommend being realistic about human vulnerability. Give away family jewelry to heirs or remove it to a bank's safety-deposit box. Don't leave wallets on desks or cash in "secret" hiding places in closets and drawers.

People with fading memories sometimes unfairly accuse paid caregivers of stealing, when they've simply forgotten where they put something. On the other hand, unfortunately, caregivers (and, by the way, some family members) do sometimes steal: a theft forced my husband's eighty-seven-year-old father to fire someone he had come to depend on. It's better to remove temptation beforehand than to find yourself continually suspicious.

BEING AN EXAMPLE

People who thrive while living with age- and health-related limitations have usually cultivated the virtues of adaptation, acceptance, and interdependence. You are never too old or weak to give and receive love, or to offer encouragement, reassurance, and praise to younger people. Don't discount the power of your example. How you conduct your life now will teach those who come after you.

The Israeli psychologist Valery Hazanov, during his training at Columbia University, learned much from the clients he worked with in New York City nursing homes. Those who did best, he noticed, were creatures of habit. One ninety-four-year-old woman whom he admired woke at 6:30 a.m. and first made her bed. Then she went for a stroll with her walker, ate breakfast, exercised in the rehabilitation room, read, ate lunch, napped, went for another walk, drank tea with a friend, ate dinner, and went to bed. Her disciplined routines gave her life structure.

"She pushes herself to do things, some of which are very difficult for her, without asking herself why it is important to do them," Hazanov wrote on Vox.com. "I think this is what keeps her alive—her movement, her pushing, *is* her life. Observing her, I have been coming to the conclusion that it might be true for all of us."

Along with structure and discipline, Hazanov noticed that joy and gratitude were crucial to residents' well-being. Those who coped best with chronic physical pain, he observed, had long been passionate about something outside themselves, something they continued to do despite age, pain, and disability. They loved spending time with a grandchild, painting watercolors, singing in a choir, or mentoring others in their profession. Developing outside passions, long before they became disabled, made tolerating reduced circumstances more bearable.

"You can't start developing the spiritual muscle when you're old," Hazanov wrote. "If you didn't *really* care about anything outside of yourself (like books, or sports, or your brother, or what is a moral life), you're not going to start when you're old and in terrible pain. Your terrible pain will be the only thing on your mind."

The very old taught Hazanov another spiritual skill: acceptance. One woman in her eighties, sitting by a window, told him: "Valery, one day you will be my age, God willing, and you will sit here, where I sit now, and you will look out of the window, as I do now. And you want to do that without regret and envy; you want to just look out at the world outside and be okay with not being a part of it anymore."

Ways to Prepare:

- Plan financially for further disability.
- Spread the caregiving burden beyond immediate family with hired help or friends. For local sources of help, call your county's Agency on Aging or dial 211.
- Ask for a referral from your primary care doctor to a physical therapist, speech therapist, or occupational therapist.
- Do everything you can to prevent a fall. Study Pilates, yoga, qigong, or t'ai chi, or take a class in fall prevention. Stay strong and get an occupational therapist to help you eliminate hazards in your home.
- If you haven't already, review and reduce medications like statins, blood pressure drugs, tranquilizers, sleeping pills, sedatives, and SSRI antidepressants.

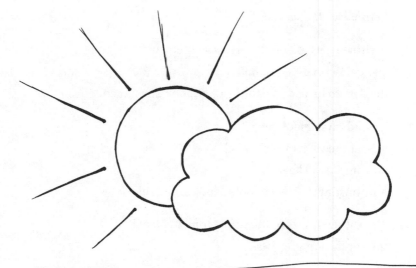

—CHAPTER 4—

Awareness of Mortality

The Art of Honest Hope • Talking to Your Doctor
Understanding the Trajectory of Your Illness
Preparing the Family • Finding Allies in Palliative Care
Reflecting on What Gives Your Life Meaning
Staying in Charge • Thinking Creatively • Redefining Hope

Perishable, It Said

Perishable, it said on the plastic container,
and below, in different ink,
the date to be used by, the last teaspoon consumed.

I found myself looking:
now at the back of each hand,
now inside the knees,
now turning over each foot to look at the sole.

Then at the leaves of the young tomato plants,
then at the arguing jays.

Under the wooden table and lifted stones, looking.
Coffee cups, olives, cheeses,
hunger, sorrow, fears—
these too would certainly vanish, without knowing when.

How suddenly then
the strange happiness took me,
like a man with strong hands and strong mouth,
inside that hour with its perishing perfumes and clashings.

—JANE HIRSHFIELD

You may find this chapter helpful if you recognize yourself (or someone you care for) in some of these statements:

- A doctor says you have a "serious" or terminal illness. This includes cancers that have reached stage four, meaning they've spread.
- An organ vital to sustaining life—your heart, brain, kidneys, lungs, or liver—is slowly failing.
- You are in the early stages of an incurable disease that worsens over time, such as amyotrophic lateral sclerosis (Lou Gehrig's disease, or ALS).
- Doctors refuse to discuss your *prognosis,* or say your disease has a *poor* or *dire* prognosis. (*Prognosis* just means a forecast of your health prospects, but in medicine it's often a euphemism for "You are approaching the end of your life.")
- Your doctors use terms like *chronic, progressive, serious, advanced, late stage* or *end stage.* (They mean incurable, worsening, worse yet, and approaching the end of life.)
- Doctors want to discuss *goals of care.* (This is medical shorthand for exploring what matters most to you, and how medicine can help you accomplish it, when time is short and cure is not in the cards.)
- You have a gut sense that following this medical appointment, your life will be forever divided into *before* and *after.*

THE ART OF HONEST HOPE

Amy Berman is a dedicated amateur artist and registered nurse who distributes health policy grants for the John A. Hartford Foundation in Manhattan. She loves to write, travel, surf, and spend time with her family, especially her grown daughter, Stephanie, with whom she shares a house in Brooklyn. One fall morning shortly after her fifty-first birthday, Amy stood in the shower and felt, on her right breast, a dimpled patch of skin the texture of orange peel and about the size of a nickel. A first round of tests revealed she had inflammatory breast cancer. Many early breast cancers are curable. But inflammatory breast cancer is a rare beast, infrequently found before it has spread.

At Maimonides Cancer Center in Brooklyn, she underwent a PET scan and a bone biopsy to explore a suspicious-looking area in her lower spine. She then scheduled a meeting with the nation's top academic expert in her cancer, at his office in a university medical center in Philadelphia.

She and her mother, Rose, who joined her from Florida, checked into a hotel and went for a walk in the rain through a neighborhood of shuttered antiques shops. They were planning to meet friends for dinner and, after the doctor's appointment the next day, go shopping for the wigs Amy would need when chemotherapy temporarily robbed her of her hair.

Amy's cell phone rang. It was her oncologist at Maimonides, calling about the biopsy. Clusters of cancer cells had been found in Amy's spine. She blurted out the news to her mother. They dropped their umbrellas and held each other as the rain poured down.

"I thought, in that moment, *I have a very short life span,*" Amy said. Her cancer had spread and would eventually kill her. Eleven to 20 percent of people with her diagnosis survive five years, and only a handful live more than seven.

Thoughts rushed through her brain. Who would guide her daughter after she was gone? How would she tell her sister, who was also her best friend? "I thought about what I was going to be giving up, about saying goodbye to people. It was a succession of overwhelmingly negative thoughts about what it means to have a terminal illness," she said. "Looking into my mother's eyes, I felt I had injured her heart, and that made me feel just that much worse."

She and her mother returned to the hotel, where Amy caught a glimpse of herself and her mother in a lobby mirror. Their faces were distraught, blotchy, and red; their eyes puffy; their cheeks slicked with tears and rain. "Seeing how I was appearing to the world shocked me into thinking, *I have decisions to make*," she said. "I turned to my mother and said, 'We need to take three deep breaths.' We took three deep breaths and burst out laughing."

Amy said to her mother, "If I spend my remaining days mourning the cancer, the cancer wins. It will take away any goodness in my life, and I refuse to allow that to happen."

They decided to go ahead and do what they would have done had there been no crisis. They returned to their rooms, put on fresh makeup, and went out to dinner with their friends. "It was a lighthearted dinner," said Amy. "It set us on a path of living and not dying."

The next morning, Amy told the famous oncologist about her biopsy results. He didn't pause. "Here's what we're going to do," he said, plowing ahead with his plan: six weeks of intense chemotherapy followed by surgery to remove her breast. Then radiation and another round of chemo.

Amy was being invited to play a role she didn't relish—that of the unquestioning patient who heroically "battles" her disease to the end. The doctor's aggressive, hail-Mary treatment plan would expose her to great suffering, and then she'd bump along—for who knew how long?—in severely damaged health. And for what? Her cancer couldn't be rooted out. She questioned the unspoken assumption that the most harrowing treatment would produce the best possible result.

The interaction was one-sided and top-down. The oncologist asked no questions. He assumed that Amy cared mainly about attacking the cancer, no matter how devastating the collateral damage to her body and her life. It was her job, apparently, to participate in a common modern medical ritual: not to question why, just to do—and then die. "There was no conversation," she said. "He was expert in everything but what really mattered to me. I thanked him for his time and left." She returned to her cancer doctor at Maimonides and never went back to Philadelphia.

Amy opted for a different rite of passage: a quiet declaration of independence. As she went forward, her doctors would be her consultants, not her bosses. She would seek out those who were curious about what mattered to her and willing to shape their treatment plans accordingly. She would weigh her medical options in the light of their impact on what the poet Mary Oliver called "your one wild and precious life." She would stay in the driver's seat. It was her life and her death.

Back at Maimonides, her original oncologist asked a more welcome question: "What do you want to accomplish?" Amy said she hoped for "Niagara Falls" trajectory: to live well for as long as possible, and then to plunge over the waterfall to death without undue delay. The oncologist suggested she start with a daily pill of Femara, which inhibits the body's production of estrogen, a stimulator of breast cancer growth. There would be no radiation, no chemo, and no mastectomy. The aim wasn't cure. It was to slow Amy's cancer while interfering as little as possible with her life.

It's been seven years since Amy stood weeping with her mother in the rain. She knows her days are numbered and she accepts it. She remains on the top side of Niagara Falls. Femara held her cancer at bay for four years before, as expected, it stopped working. She's now on a second estrogen-inhibiting pill, tamoxifen, which she expects to be effective for about half as long as Femara was. She takes another drug to keep her bones strong and to fend off the osteoporosis that is a by-product of tamoxifen. She finds other side effects—prematurely aging skin, energy loss after taking her pills at night, and high temperatures that feel like sustained hot flashes—acceptable in light of her hunger for continued life.

She's never spent an afternoon in a recliner while a toxic chemotherapy dripped into her veins. She's never been hospitalized, or been too weak to drive, or needed a home health aide. Her hair hasn't fallen out. She hasn't gone into debt. She has climbed the Great Wall of China, ridden a jet ski to the base of the Statue of Liberty, and seen her daughter, Stephanie, graduate from college and get married. She has made quality of life her priority, and paradoxically she's outlived many people who opt for more grueling treatments. "Most doctors," she says, "focus only on length of life. That's not my only metric."

We are all mortal. But knowing this abstractly and feeling it viscerally are not the same. The bad news may arrive as a stunning diagnosis, or more ambiguously and unpredictably, as a vital organ slowly fails. Sometimes incurable illnesses (and their treatments) create long periods of disability, necessitating immediate plans to get caregivers and support teams in place. Others permit months to years of continued high functioning.

People who do well in this health stage have usually mastered the tricky art of accepting death while continuing to live. They decide what matters to them and make their medical choices according to their own lights. They do what they love. They expand the boundaries of the word "hope" to encompass miracles beyond cure, such as family reconciliation, leaving their survivors in good shape, or taking the grandkids on one last memorable trip to Disneyland. They often get support from a relatively new medical specialty: palliative care. This misunderstood approach focuses on relieving suffering, improving day-to-day well-being and functioning, and helping patients make medical choices in alignment with what matters most to them.

TALKING TO YOUR DOCTOR

In modern health care, doctors sometimes deliver bad news and then barely pause before proposing (or simply informing you of) their plan for your treatment. I suggest you stop and take a breath after receiving a tough diagnosis. Most forms of modern death move slowly. There is no harm in taking a few days to tend to the soul, to let awareness sink in, to talk with friends, and to gather information before deciding how you want to proceed. Going forward you will need clear information, support in grieving your losses, and time to reflect on new ways to define hope.

"You almost become numb," said Ron Belcher, who was seventy-two and had severe congestive heart failure when he was told that his colonoscopy had revealed early signs of colon cancer. Much to his surprise, his surgeon bluntly recommended against surgery. His cancer, she said, was slow-growing; he was more likely to die *with* it than *of* it. Given the stress of the operation and the severity of his heart problems, she said, he had a 90 percent chance of dying within two months if he had surgery.

"You say to yourself, okay, I gotta process this, but I can't process this right now," Ron said. "I'm in front of a group of doctors and a daughter-in-law who's also had cancer. I've got to go home and meditate, think about this in private, mull my options, and cry if I need to cry." Ron took a week to discuss the pros and cons with his family and decided against surgery. "I appreciated that my surgeon didn't beat around the bush," he said, "but it was the most gut-wrenching decision I ever had to make."

Find people capable of listening to you without judgment—be it a friend, relative, or hospital social worker or chaplain. Most health systems offer support groups for people with terminal illnesses, and there you may find a welcoming community that can address every dimension of your experience—not just your medical decisions, but your emotional, practical, and spiritual concerns. People who go to support groups tend to be less stressed and better informed than those who don't attend them, and sometimes they live longer.

After awareness and acceptance comes action. When you feel capable, it's time to hold an honest, difficult, conversation with your doctor. These talks can be so painful that most doctors and patients simply don't have them. But they are vital if you want to lay continued claim to your life and your death. Ariadne Labs in Boston, founded by the surgeon-author Atul Gawande, is doing the critical work of training doctors in how to hold these conversations, as is oncologist Anthony Back, of the University of Washington, at Vitaltalk. But until training improves, "physicians are waiting for the patient to bring things up and patients are waiting for the physicians to bring them up," says Alvin H. "Woody" Moss, MD, a kidney specialist and palliative care doctor at the University of West Virginia's medical school. "There's a conspiracy of silence." Break it.

In one study of patients with fatal lung cancers, half hadn't discussed hospice with their doctors two months before their deaths, and in another, three-quarters of patients with incurable, meta-static lung cancer had the mistaken impression that cure was possible. As Moss puts it bluntly, "Doctors usually sugarcoat how bad things are."

If you can, bring a friend or relative to the meeting to provide emotional support, take notes, and ask follow-up questions. Amy Berman recommends that you open with some version of "I want a realistic picture, so I can plan." If the answers you get are filled with incomprehensible medicalese, I suggest you try some version of "I don't understand. Would you say that again, more simply?" And if you get a clear answer, it's great to say, "Thank you, that is exactly what I was looking for!"

Some physicians worry that telling you the truth will take away your hope. But knowledge is empowering. People with a clear understanding of the courses of their illnesses tend to do as well or better physically than those kept in the dark, and they don't suffer any more or less emotional distress. "Some people don't want to know what the future holds," says Ron Hoffman, the founder of Compassionate Care ALS (Lou Gehrig's disease) in Falmouth, Massachusetts, who has supported hundreds of people through the last stages of their lives. "But on the whole, those who are willing to explore and navigate the terrain of their mortality have more peaceful, gentle, and even beautiful deaths."

Some people get angry when their doctors deliver bad news bluntly. But consider, for a moment, the alternative. One nurse, assigned to improve treatment of the terminally ill in her large health system's emergency rooms, told me of encountering "staggering numbers of patients with devastating symptoms of stage four cancers who were told they were dying by [an emergency room] physician who did not know them." They were shocked by the news and sent home to die under hospice care, making it unlikely they'd ever again see, or say goodbye to, the oncologist with whom they'd developed a trusting relationship.

"These patients often feel abandoned at their greatest moment of need," she went on. "But we have not been successful in working with the oncologists to have honest discussions earlier, because the oncologists tell us their patients fire them if they are truthful."

UNDERSTANDING THE TRAJECTORY OF YOUR ILLNESS

Go ahead and ask. Make sure you understand the trajectory of your illness if it follows its usual course. If you have cancer, get clear on its stage and its type in the context of your age and overall health, which will shape your trajectory. Some cancers are curable and others, including almost all stage four cancers (despite recent advances in immunotherapy) are not. Some move slowly and, with treatment, permit years of high functioning, and others usually kill within a year. Precise predictions of the time you have left are rarely accurate, and doctors, on average, overestimate their patients' survival time by four to six times. You can, however, get a rough estimate of whether you have "days, weeks, months, or years." That is meaningful enough to frame your choices.

Take a step further. Ask not only about length of life, but about how you will feel and function, and how proposed treatments may affect your well-being. You may need to find caregivers or a health care agent, to sign an advance directive, to buy adaptive equipment, or to apply for Social Security disability or other public benefits. You may choose to say no to drugs and procedures with severe side effects and dubious payoffs. Or, if you know that a treatment will be debilitating, you may seize the bittersweet gift of time to first take a photography class or visit relatives, or to reconcile with an estranged family member.

Improving your understanding and command of the situation can reduce feelings of helplessness, and give people who love you specific ways to help. If your doctor refuses to discuss your prognosis at all—and some do—consider that a warning sign. You are unlikely to feel empowered if you are left in the dark. If, after a try or two, you still have only the foggiest picture, I suggest you find a new specialist who is more forthcoming, or add a palliative care doctor to your team, as explained on page 90. As a supplement, the American Cancer Society offers accurate information online, and so does the Mayo Clinic. (Beware, however, of sites primarily funded by pharmaceutical companies and others that are trying to sell you something.)

Many people find that a pen-and-paper sketch helps them visualize what the future holds. Below are four common trajectories to the end of life. Three of them (Niagara Falls, Looping Decline, and The Dwindles) were first formulated in 2005 by the pioneering geriatrician Joanne Lynn and were included in 2014 in Atul Gawande's bestselling book *Being Mortal*. The stair step pathway was first sketched for me by a counselor for the Alzheimer's Association.

You might ask your doctor which best fits your situation, and if none do, ask him or her to draw you another.

The Niagara Falls Trajectory

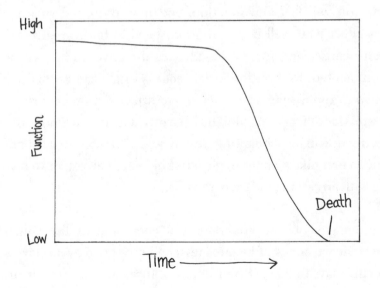

This pathway is marked by months to years of high functioning, followed by a rapid decline of a few weeks or months. It is common in kidney failure without dialysis and in cancers treated once or twice. When symptoms are well managed, thanks to palliative care or hospice programs, people often can continue to work, do things they enjoy, and even go out for coffee with friends until a few weeks before death.

Looping Decline

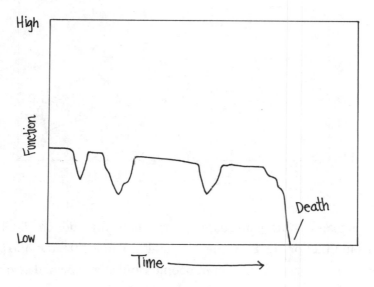

Repeated health crises land people in the hospital, where they recover somewhat and return home, only to decline until the next crisis. It's hard to precisely predict death, as there's no way of knowing which hospitalization will turn out to be the final one. This trajectory is common during the failure of vital organs, in heart and lung diseases that often strike in the seventies and eighties, and in cancers at any age treated repeatedly with chemotherapy and radiation with strong side effects. People need help with daily chores, at first occasionally and then frequently. Some crises can be averted with physician house calls and close medical management. Death sometimes comes after a final catastrophe, and sometimes after a patient tires of repeated treatment or says something like "no more hospitals."

Stair Step Down

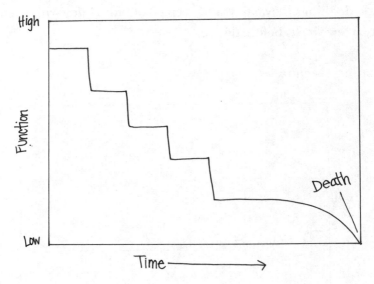

Long and short plateaus are punctuated by sudden, drastic drops in functioning. Each "new normal" is worse than the one before. This pattern is common in people who have repeated strokes or vascular dementia, and in the old and frail who undergo repeated hospitalizations that set off delirium (hallucinations and prolonged cognitive confusion) or otherwise inadvertently cause harm.

The Dwindles

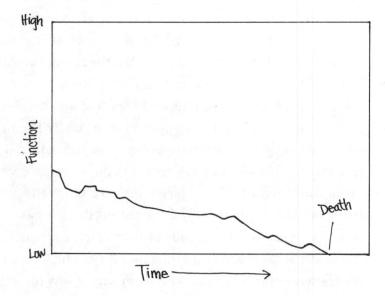

Strength and vitality fade away, along with appetite and interest in living. Small maladies accumulate, senses fail, muscles weaken, and over time the body just wears out. The need for help with daily life may last as long as a decade. This trajectory is common in dementia, extreme old age, and kidney failure with dialysis. Medical decisions often fall to family members. Death sometimes comes naturally and gently, or after a decision to forgo antibiotics or otherwise let nature take its course. At other times, death arrives in the form of a pneumonia, a broken hip, or an infection that would not have vanquished a hardier person.

PREPARING THE FAMILY

Share your sketches with your family. It takes time for people to absorb the notion that you will die someday, and the unprepared can wreak havoc at the end of life. Keep talking until everyone accepts the truth. Doctors say that it's often a conflicted family member who insists on risky, last-ditch treatments. The doctors go along because they fear lawsuits, complaints, and bad professional reviews. "I can't begin to tell you the times I did not want to operate on someone because it was futile or because the quality of their remaining time would greatly suffer," one surgeon told me. "But the family were absolutely dead set and insisted on 'everything being done.'

"Sure, I could refuse and recommend they find another doctor, but if the patient dies in the meantime, I come under fire and 'review' even if I believe that *not* intervening is the right thing. If a family even tries to file a lawsuit, it stays with a physician's record." So she reluctantly performs Hail Mary surgeries after, as she puts it, "covering my butt" by thoroughly documenting that she has disclosed the risks. This sometimes ends with watching a patient die a horrible death, sedated and on a ventilator. "It's painful for me to see and experience this," she said, "since I am part of why (despite not wanting to be) the patient is not having a dignified death."

FINDING ALLIES IN PALLIATIVE CARE

Once you understand the general contours of what you're facing, I recommend you add a palliative care doctor to your team. Many people have never heard of palliative care, or else confuse it with hospice, but don't let that stop you. (Briefly, hospice is for people likely to die within six months, while palliative care is helpful much earlier in the course of a long illness.) Every dimension of your experience will probably be easier with this extra layer of support.

Palliative care focuses primarily on relieving suffering and improving function, not on curing disease. The word "palliative" has been a recognized part of medicine since at least 1543, when the first English translation of an earlier treatise by the Venetian doctor Giovanni da Vigo appeared, recommending *"apalliating"* incurable illnesses by "gentle remedies" rather than attacking a disease at its root. It became a distinct medical specialty in the 1970s, when other branches of medicine started to focus almost exclusively on prolonging life. It has become the preeminent medical ally for anyone who wants to live a good life while coping with a debilitating illness.

In some health systems palliative care is called prehospice, supportive care, pain management, symptom management, comfort care, or serious or advanced illness management. No matter what it's called, you should ask for it: palliative care improves well-being and survival times so significantly that both the American Heart Association and the American Society of Clinical Oncology recommend it as early as possible.

Unlike hospice, which is usually reimbursed by insurance only when people abandon all attempts at cure and are within six months of dying, you can get palliative care while you are still fighting disease and hope to live much longer. Its doctors and nurses will work alongside your cure-oriented specialists. Like physical and occupational therapists, they won't focus so much on "what's the matter *with* you." Instead, they will ask "what matters *to* you" and help you achieve it. They are experts at managing fatigue, nausea, anxiety, and breathlessness. They also step in as truth-tellers, counselors, and medical-decision coaches when other doctors feel unequipped to play those roles. They are not afraid to talk frankly about the realities of death and disability, and to help you prepare for them emotionally and practically. And because they work in teams and focus on the needs of the whole person, they often save people from falling through the cracks in fragmented health systems.

Recent research has shown that people who get palliative care have fewer health crises and spend less time in hospitals, and are therefore less often exposed to medical errors and infections. They die in hospitals less frequently, and enroll in hospice earlier. They experience less pain and suffering and they tend to leave their survivors in greater emotional peace. And oddly enough, they often live longer than people who continue with harsh, last-ditch, supposedly life-prolonging treatments.

———

Palliative care saved Amy Berman a great deal of unnecessary suffering when she developed excruciating pain in her back, four years after her cancer diagnosis. Cancer cells had migrated from her spine to her lower ribs, inflaming nerve endings. The standard treatment was ten to twenty doses of radiation, administered once a day for two to four weeks. The predicted side effects included exhaustion, hair loss, blistered skin, nerve damage, and a temporarily weakened immune system.

Before proceeding, Amy consulted with a palliative care specialist at Maimonides to weigh her pros, cons, and alternatives. Together they found studies showing that a single carefully focused burst of more intense radiation would work as well as multiple weaker blasts. That's what Amy chose—after a struggle with her insurance company, which at first didn't want to pay for the expensive scan necessary to deliver the radiation safely. Her back pain disappeared in one day, saving her pain, lost work time, and hundreds if not thousands of dollars in insurance co-pays.

REFLECTING ON WHAT GIVES YOUR LIFE MEANING

A palliative care doctor helped Jerry Romano, a textbook editor in Menlo Park, California, who had to retire in his sixties after a heart attack and open-heart surgery. By the time he turned seventy, his heart problems had become so bad that his cardiologist arranged for an implanted defibrillator. Sometimes called "an emergency room in your chest," defibrillators deliver massive and painful shocks to the heart to "reboot" it if it starts beating so erratically that life is threatened. (Less intrusive pacemakers, by contrast, keep hearts beating at a healthy, regular rhythm by delivering consistent, tiny electric pulses that are imperceptible to the patient.) The device did nothing for Jerry's symptoms, chest pain and breathlessness, which kept him from doing what gave his life meaning—making beautiful painted wooden airplanes and toys for children in his backyard woodshop. Tired of a life that had lost its savor, he asked to have his defibrillator deactivated. After this was done, a palliative care doctor put him on oxygen at night (relieving his breathlessness) and adjusted his medications (easing his chest pain). He returned to his woodshop to build toys, and once again he felt life was worth living.

If your specialist balks and says it's "too early" for a referral to palliative care (unfortunately this is still a common response) please note that in some health systems, you can call the palliative care department directly without a doctor's referral. Some hospices also provide palliative care, and they can often help you find practitioners who provide it, as can the website getpalliativecare.org.

If you can't find palliative care, do what its doctors would do: make sure you articulate what makes your life worth living, and see that the treatment you get serves those goals. "Do you like to go to the opera?" asks Dawn Gross, MD, a palliative care specialist at the University of California medical school in San Francisco. "Do you want to be able to garden, or sing, or play the piano, do the crossword puzzle, ski, go shopping, or be able to eat or talk to your grandkids?" Know what gives you joy, and let your doctors know, at every visit, whether you can still do it.

"A doctor will not be thinking in terms of whether you can garden," Gross said. "They'll just be thinking, 'I'm going to do whatever I can to slow this down and come as close to curing it as I can.' If you don't have a really good footing, you will get sucked into a powerful current within medicine that assumes that you want to try to live forever, no matter what."

At each visit, remind your doctor (and perhaps yourself) what matters to you. "When a patient tells me that they were able to paint or make the bed, that's incredibly helpful to me," says Anthony Back, a leading oncologist at the University of Washington who helped found a program called Vitaltalk, which trains oncologists in how to hold meaningful conversations with patients. "It's very different from reporting your symptoms on a ten-point scale."

Finally, address your fears. Ask your doctor:

- What is it like to die of my disease, and how can medicine ease my symptoms?
- Will you still be my doctor if I decide to opt for strictly palliative care?
- When do patients with my disease benefit most from enrolling in hospice?

STAYING IN CHARGE

Don't let the business of medicine eclipse the business of living. Spend your limited energy and time on things that matter to you. To that end, feel free to turn down tests, treatments, and doctor's visits that don't serve your purposes. Dr. Back suggests asking your doctor, "How is this test going to change what we're doing—or are we just doing it for more information? If that's the case, I'd just as soon skip it."

You have no obligation to create a voluminous medical history or to monitor a condition that can't be cured. Shrinking a tumor or stopping it from growing sounds good. But oddly enough, tumor shrinkage in and of itself doesn't predict an extended life span or improved day-to-day well-being. Between 2004 and 2014, about 74 percent of cancer drugs approved by the FDA as "effective" because they arrested tumor growth did not improve patient's survival time by a single day. (Ask, instead, if the treatment is "clinically effective," meaning that it actually benefits patients.) Resist focusing on repeated scans, and check in with your own body. How well you feel, and how much or little you can do, are more meaningful measures of your health and better predictors of what your future holds.

Don't, by the way, place much stock in media hype about breakthroughs around the corner. They've been appearing regularly for half a century. Take for instance, recent advances in immunotherapy for cancer. A small group of people get an extended plateau, but immunotherapy is not, so far, a cure. What is rarely discussed is that after a "honeymoon period" when tumors melt away, the cancer usually returns. Overall time gained is often limited to a few months, and the treatment's suppression of the immune system produces terrible side effects that can be health-destroying and even life-ending.

Some treatments forestall death for years with relatively gentle side effects. Others delay death without restoring health. Still others are triple losers: they damage the quality of remaining life, they reduce its length, and they cost a fortune in co-pays. This medical labyrinth is confusing even to people, like Amy Berman, with substantial medical training.

As a guide to this confusing environment, keep in mind the law of diminishing returns. If your disease is terminal, each successive round of treatment is likely to produce fewer gains, and to work for a shorter time, than the one before it. This is especially true if you are growing weaker. In lung cancer, average survival time is four months after a third "line," or round of treatment. The fourth line produces no better results than no treatment at all and, in the words of oncologist and palliative care doctor Thomas Smith of Johns Hopkins, is "ineffective, toxic, and delays hospice use."

Therefore, keep making sure you understand how your life, functioning, and well-being will be affected by a demanding treatment, be it repeated chemotherapy, an external heart pump, or dialysis. Many of these are called "halfway technologies" because they ward off death without restoring health. They often place massive burdens on caregivers and substantially damage the quality of remaining life. Just because a doctor offers something, and insurance will pay for it, doesn't make it a good idea. Sometimes doctors are secretly relieved when patients reject a harrowing treatment with minimal payoffs that they felt duty bound to offer. You are not required, legally or morally, to agree to any procedure you don't want. Most people believe that there are fates worse than death, and it's up to you to decide where *you* draw that line.

As you proceed, keep making sure that you and your doctor remain on the same page. Each time a new treatment is proposed, ask your doctor what he or she hopes to accomplish. As a reminder, the five traditional duties of medicine are: to prevent disease; to restore functioning; to prolong life; to relieve suffering; and to attend the dying. Sometimes these goals are in sync; toward the end of life they can be at cross-purposes. Which goal is your doctor trying to fulfill? Ask: "Do you hope this will give me more time? Cure my disease, or slow it down? Improve how I feel or function day to day?" Then think through whether these priorities match your own, and whether the trade-offs are worthwhile to you.

It may help you retain your agency and your moral authority if you understand that financial incentives, hidden from your view, promote overtreatment. The pharmaceutical industry alone has more than three thousand lobbyists in Washington who shape health policy to their clients' advantages. Few people with cancer know, for instance, that oncologists get more than half of their revenue from markups (in 2017, of 4.3 percent) that they are allowed to add to the price of the chemotherapy drugs they prescribe and administer. This funding system, known as "buy and bill," creates an unfortunate incentive to prescribe the most expensive chemo and to infuse it long after it stops being helpful. This peculiar system underpays oncologists for making time for difficult conversations, and puts them all in a terrible bind.

So stay in the driver's seat. Make the best decisions you can in light of uncertainty and your gut sense of what you can tolerate. "I've been in many support groups through the years," said Merijane Block, who lived for two decades with a slow-moving metastatic breast cancer that eventually spread to her spine. "I've seen women who did everything . . . and they died. I've known women who couldn't bring themselves to do everything . . . and they died. It's one big crapshoot."

Merijane underwent radiation, surgeries, and drug treatments. But for twenty years, she refused chemotherapies that would have been infused directly into her bloodstream and damaged noncancerous tissues in her skin, hair, and bone marrow. "I just couldn't take a medicine that destroys healthy cells and causes so much devastation," she said. "I had a very strong feeling it would kill either my body or my soul."

Over time her cancer, in tandem with the radiation she was given to slow its progress, left Merijane in chronic pain. She used a walker and then a wheelchair. "The days of the somewhat-easier drugs appear to be over for me," she said. Fearing the prospect of a painful, drawn-out death, she met with a palliative care doctor at her medical center.

He coached her on how to have a frank talk with her oncologist, a "brilliant clinician" with whom Merijane had bonded, but found intimidating. At their next meeting, Merijane put her hand on top of her oncologist's hand and said to her gently, "The time is going to come when I'm going to shift to strictly palliative care. Will you still be able to be my doctor?" The oncologist's eyes filled with tears. She said, "I'll be with you till the end," and both women began crying.

When a disease continues to advance, some people pin their hopes on becoming an experimental subject in a clinical trial of an untested drug. I suggest that before you enter a "stage one clinical trial," you think hard about your motives. Some people find meaning in contributing to scientific knowledge before they die, and that is an achievable goal. But being a guinea pig in a clinical trial is a gamble with miniscule odds of improving your health or extending your life.

Consider the statistics. The FDA never approves 95 percent of untested cancer drugs that begin clinical trials, because they prove to be either dangerous, or ineffective, or both. According to a groundbreaking study in the *New England Journal of Medicine,* only 5 percent of volunteer subjects gained more time. Of those who did, half (2.5 percent of the total) lived less than an additional six months, and there are no good studies assessing the quality of that time. Some participants suffer side effects so severe that they drop out of the study or die sooner, with more suffering, than they would have otherwise. This dismal record recently led the medical ethicist Jonathan Kimmelman to write, in the *Journal of Clinical Oncology,* that it was time to deflate "the unscrupulous marketing of unproven interventions to desperate patients."

So think through what a clinical trial asks of you. When time is short, do you want to spend it at clinic appointments? "Energy is your most precious commodity," says oncologist Anthony Back. "Think about where you want to spend it. People think of clinical trials as risk-free lottery tickets, but they have their price."

THINKING CREATIVELY

For some people, throwing "everything but the kitchen sink" at a fatal illness has become a medical rite of passage. In the words of the noted cancer researcher and physician Siddhartha Mukherjee, author of *The Emperor of All Maladies,* this approach can lead to "a scorched-earth operation with many long-term consequences." There's an unspoken belief, widely held among patients and doctors, that the more tests, procedures, specialists, treatments, and hospital visits you undergo, the longer and better you will live. But it can be just the opposite. For both the fragile and the relatively robust in their last months of living with cancer, new research is strongly suggesting that more chemotherapy frequently shortens life and contributes to a worse quality of death.

Much scientific research investigates treatments that attack diseases head-on. Less research explores how the body fights off disease. Cancerous tumors, Mukherjee notes, shed thousands of cells into the bloodstream daily, but only in some people do those cells develop into metastases. I encourage you to explore the many low-cost, low-risk ways you can strengthen your immune system, your first line of defense. They might improve how you feel and function today and are unlikely to do you harm. I'm not suggesting that you substitute carrot juice for a lumpectomy if you have a treatable breast cancer, but simply that you honor the capacity of your body, and your mind, to contribute to your healing.

Studies observing large groups of patients suggest that people with life-limiting illnesses who exercise, adopt a healthy diet, and get emotional support—as a complement, not a substitute, for conventional medicine—tend to live longer. A protein-sparing vegan diet can slow kidney failure. People with high bloodstream levels of vitamin D tend to do better after treatment for colon cancer. So do those adopting a so-called non-Western diet like the Mediterranean Diet, substituting vegetables, whole grains, olive oil, fish, and fruit for red meat, sugar, white bread, and other heavily processed "food products." Acupuncture can reduce all sorts of pain. Stick with complementary remedies that are gentle, unlikely to hurt you, and may prove helpful. Most will not be reimbursed by Medicare or other insurance.

Marijuana for medical purposes, now legal in twenty-nine states, has been used in the West since at least 1850, when Ada Lovelace, the pioneering English mathematician and daughter of Lord Byron, used it to relieve the pain of her terminal cancer. Some palliative care physicians prescribe marijuana extracts containing high levels of THC (tetrahydrocannabinol) and say they improve appetite, and control pain and nausea better, than prescription pharmaceuticals—with the enjoyable side effect of euphoria. Hemp-derived oils saturated with the more staid psychoactive compound CBD or cannabidiol (a less mind-bending component of marijuana and hemp which is not on the federal government's list of controlled substances) are widely available online without prescription. CBD is reported to relieve pain and anxiety without producing the euphoria of THC, but it doesn't improve appetite.

REDEFINING HOPE

"I am not a huge fan of hope," says oncologist Tony Back. He urges his patients not to concentrate so hard on hopes that they forget about today. "A lot of people want to finish something," he says. "They want to end up in some kind of peace, or to reconnect with people in some way. If only they could orient themselves to enjoy what is happening in the moment!" He also urges them to think about this question: "What is something you could do *today* that you could really enjoy?"

Below are some hopes, and some rites of passage, to consider, in place of a futile war on death:

Leave a good emotional legacy. In anticipation of death, some people write "legacy letters" to their children and grandchildren, describing what life has taught them. Others write milestone letters for daughters and sons to open on the day of a college graduation or wedding. "To be there when a son or daughter has a first child—that may not be an achievable goal," says Shoshana Helman, a palliative care doctor at Kaiser Permanente in Redwood City, California. "But writing a letter that can be opened at that time is achievable."

Enjoy the time you have left. When Ted Marshall, a fine carpenter trained in traditional Japanese joinery, learned he had the deadly brain tumor glioblastoma, he and his wife, Sharry, threw everything possible into the path of his cancer: surgery, radiation, conventional chemotherapies and off-label drugs, oriental medicine, a low-carbohydrate diet, a skull cap that zaps tumors with electrical currents, and blue scorpion venom from Cuba.

They also talked openly about how they wanted to live if Ted had six months to two years left. Sharry wanted him to be as happy as possible. Ted wanted to finish renovating the apartment they'd bought in a cooperative housing community in Richmond, California, so that he'd leave Sharry housed and in good financial shape.

The couple took as their motto "Don't postpone joy." In the first year, they went to a cowboy poetry gathering in Elko, Nevada; a fiddle festival in Port Townsend, Washington; and American "roots music" gatherings in Asheville, North Carolina, and Clifftop, West Virginia. After their return, Ted finished remodeling the couple's home with the help of friends. "We did a good job," Sharry said, "of wringing every drop of fun we could out of the life he had left."

Over the next three years, Ted gradually lost the ability to spell, to work, to drive, and to remember to close the refrigerator. Nothing about it was easy, but he died peacefully at the age of sixty-eight, under hospice care, in the couple's beautifully renovated, mortgage-free home.

Go on an adventure. Norma Jean Bauerschmidt, a retired nurse of ninety living in Presque Isle, Michigan, refused a hysterectomy and chemotherapy after learning she had stage four uterine cancer. She declined to enter a nursing home and instead moved into an RV with her son and daughter-in-law. The trio spent a year visiting national parks, with Norma moving about at first on foot, then in a wheelchair, and ultimately with the help of an oxygen tank. Instead of undergoing CAT scans, Norma got her first pedicure, mounted a horse, and rode in a hot-air balloon.

A month before her death, her son parked the RV on a friend's land in Friday Harbor, on Whidbey Island off the coast of Seattle, and Norma enrolled in hospice care. She was ninety-one when she died, thirteen months after setting out on the road.

Leave loved ones in good shape. Amy Berman and her daughter, Stephanie, have updated the house they share, choosing paint colors and finishes in Stephanie's taste—"so it can feel like hers when I'm gone," as Amy said. Her daughter currently writes the checks for the household bills, so she won't be at sea after her mother dies. Mother and daughter frequently get together with extended family, to ensure that Stephanie will feel known, protected, and loved in the future.

Amy keeps a notebook with detailed information about how to handle her finances and run the household when she is alive but no longer able to manage. She's written notes about her gravesite, whom to call after she dies, and even where to order the food for the gathering after her memorial service. Her bank account will roll over to Stephanie automatically on her death, and so will her 401K.

"These acts may sound mundane but they are all deep acts of acceptance of my mortality and my focus on those I will leave behind," Amy said. "They're selfless acts of love, even if they seem trivial."

Amy doesn't have strong preferences for her funeral, as she thinks its purpose is to comfort the living. But she expects that her daughter will follow traditional Jewish mourning rituals, beginning with sitting shiva—staying home with mirrors covered and a candle burning for seven days while receiving visits from friends who bring food and share memories of her mother. Stephanie will recite the mourners kaddish, a short daily prayer glorifying God, for eleven months. On the one-year anniversary of Amy's death, and every year thereafter, Stephanie will light a *yahrzeit* anniversary candle, which will burn for twenty-four hours before the flame dies out. Also on the first anniversary, Amy said, "My daughter will do an unveiling of my headstone as the closure on her grieving. When she visits my grave in future years, she will find a stone to leave on my headstone."

All that is in the future. For the present, Amy says, "I don't think about myself as dying. I am living until proven otherwise and I choose to live fully." You don't need a fatal diagnosis to live with this double awareness.

Ways to Prepare:

- Pause before making any major medical decisions.
- Join a support group.
- Find a palliative care doctor or nurse.

Break the silence and ask your doctor questions, including:

- Can you sketch the usual trajectory of my illness?
- What do you hope this treatment will do for me?
- How will it affect how I feel day to day?
- What are the pros, cons, and alternatives?
- What is it like to die of my disease, and how can medicine ease my symptoms?
- Will you still be my doctor if I opt for strictly palliative care?
- When do patients with my disease benefit most from hospice?

Ask yourself:

- What activities or capacities make my life worth living?
- What are my greatest fears and regrets?
- Given that time may be short, how do I want to spend it?

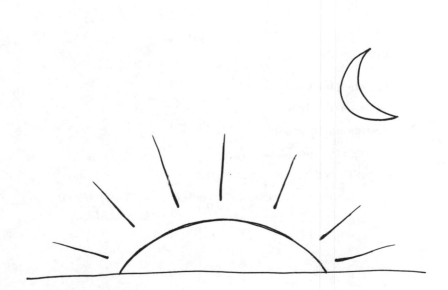

CHAPTER 5

House of Cards

If Only Someone Had Warned Us • Recognizing Frailty
Avoiding the Hospital • Finding Allies in House Call Programs
Upgrading Advance Directives • Coping with Dementia
Shifting to Comfort Care • Enjoying Your Red Velvet Cake

Although the Wind . . .

Although the wind
blows terribly here,
the moonlight also leaks
between the roof planks
of this ruined house.

—IZUMI SHIKIBU, translated by JANE HIRSHFIELD
and MARIKO ARATANI

You are likely to find this chapter helpful if you recognize yourself, or someone you care for, in some of the following statements. Because many frail people have some dementia and are no longer making their own medical decisions, I am addressing this chapter not only to people in this stage, but to their caregivers.

- You have (or someone you love has) "the dwindles": zest for living is melting away, along with appetite, energy, and investment in relationships.
- It takes you more than twenty seconds to rise from a chair, walk ten feet at a normal pace, turn around, walk back, and sit down. (This alone is a classic indicator of frailty: try it with a timer.)
- You've lost ten pounds, or 10 percent of body weight, within the past year.
- You can't walk half a mile unaided, unscrew a jar, or pick up a dining room chair.
- To get up, you push up with both hands.
- You fall frequently, have "graduated" to a walker or a wheelchair, or use tabletops and counters for balance.
- You spend ten hours or more a day sleeping.
- You need help from hired caregivers, or you live in a nursing home, in assisted living, or with relatives.
- You've gone to the emergency room at least once in the past year, and come back worse, not better.
- You have progressed from forgetting names to forgetting the way home.

IF ONLY SOMEONE HAD WARNED US

Daniel Hoefer, MD, is the chief medical director for hospice, outpatient palliative care, and other serious illness programs for the Sharp Rees-Stealy Health System, a huge nonprofit HMO in San Diego. He sometimes tells his older patients to imagine their bodies as bank accounts. From the twenties through the late forties, he says, these physiological accounts overflow with energy and resilience. With all that vitality to draw on, people recover quickly and well from accidents, illnesses, and surgeries.

But the energy storehouse of the human body is finite. From late middle age to advanced old age, we draw down our reserves. The immune system weakens, degenerative diseases afflict vital organs, muscles wither, nerves die off, and recovery from any blow takes longer. In time, the bank account runs out. Then any trauma—a fall, an accident, even a well-intentioned but stressful medical procedure—can have disastrous consequences.

Take, for instance, what happened to Daniel's father.

Rick Hoefer was a navy veteran and retired airline pilot who, as a young man, loved to play the clarinet and ride motorcycles. He lived with his wife, Marie, in Mission Viejo, a tree-lined suburb in Orange County about two hours' drive from Daniel's home in San Diego. The Hoefers had lived on the same street for forty years. It was a place where neighbors looked out for each other.

Rick celebrated his eightieth birthday with his mind still clear. He socialized with his four grown children and loved to watch his grandchildren play in his pool. But he was coping with general age-related decline, compounded by three other serious coexisting health conditions: diabetes, heart disease, and a low-red-blood-cell problem. He slept ten to twelve hours a day. He didn't go out much and he used a walker to shuffle from room to room.

He was, as Daniel put it, "toting along, doing okay," living quasi-independently with help from his wife and neighbors and sporadic check-ins from Daniel and his three siblings. Then, when Rick was eighty-three, Daniel noticed that his father's ankles were swollen with fluid, often a sign of heart trouble. A cardiologist discovered that Rick's aortic valve was narrowed, limiting his heart's ability to pump effectively. The doctor recommended an innovative procedure known as a TAVR (trans aortic valve replacement). A TAVR involves floating an artificial valve down an artery and popping it into place remotely, without cutting into the chest. It is often suggested for people too old and frail to withstand classic open-heart surgery.

Daniel Hoefer had spent decades caring for frail older people. He worried that his father didn't have the reserves to bounce back from a TAVR. Looked at one by one, each of his father's health problems seemed manageable. But in combination, they were more troubling.

In a talk he gives to other doctors, entitled "If Only Someone Had Warned Us," Hoefer reminds his fellow doctors of the many studies showing that frail patients are more likely to suffer complications, to stay in the hospital longer, and to be discharged to skilled nursing after surgery rather than returned home.

Even for the young and robust, hospitals can be not only uncomfortable, but dangerous. More than a quarter of a million Americans die annually from hospital errors, such as hospital-acquired infections and medication mix-ups. Such mistakes are the nation's third leading cause of death, and frail people are less likely to survive them. The frail are also more vulnerable to ordinary hospital stresses, like noise, unhealthy food, nighttime interruptions for the taking of vital signs, and long periods of inactivity.

Thanks to recent reforms, hospitals and surgeons are carefully tracked and rated harshly by government agencies if their patients fall in the hospital, don't survive for thirty days after surgery, pick up an infection, or are rehospitalized within thirty days of release. But nobody tracks whether those same patients lose their memories or their ability to walk, or have to move permanently to a nursing home after a hospital stay. Few, outside the family, will even know.

Which explains why Daniel's concern was so simple. His father's heart might function better after the procedure. But the human being containing the heart might function worse.

Daniel sent his father medical studies and peppered him with questions. Had the cardiologist discussed surgical risks "in the context of your frailty"? Under the best of circumstances, the TAVR carried a 14 percent chance of a serious complication, such as a stroke, heart attack, severe bleeding, or kidney damage. Rick's doctor did in fact discuss those risks, but he didn't foresee the possibility of catastrophic, global, mental, or physical decline.

Rick thanked his son for his concerns. He and his cardiologist settled on a less invasive outpatient procedure, called a "balloon valvuloplasty," to stretch open his stiff aortic valve.

In a hospital cardiac catheterization lab, doctors floated a soft thin tube down a blood vessel to Rick's heart and then inflated a balloon to widen the valve and improve blood flow. Rick didn't spend a single night in the hospital. His heart pumped more efficiently and the extra fluid came off his legs like magic. According to the standards by which surgeons, hospitals, and government agencies judge success, the procedure was a success.

But not for Rick. Everything Daniel feared came true.

It wasn't a heart attack, stroke, or a medical error that undid his father. It wasn't even a prolonged hospital stay. It was a cascade of inflammatory reactions to stress, affecting many bodily systems, including Rick's brain. Before the valvuloplasty Rick had slept ten to twelve hours a day. Afterward, he slept sixteen, and then twenty. Beforehand, he'd been alert and involved with life. He came home from the procedure exhausted, disoriented, inattentive, and sometimes delirious. He stayed confused for three weeks.

Rick Hoefer rarely thought with clarity again. He had hallucinations at night that frightened his wife.

Older people lose a stunning 5 percent of their muscle mass each day they lie in bed. After three weeks of inactivity, Rick's withered legs were little more than bone covered by paper-thin skin. He was too weak to sit up in a chair. Before, he'd trundled on his walker from room to room. Now it took two people to get him out of bed and into a wheelchair. He never walked again.

Prior to the valvuloplasty, Daniel's father could have been knocked over by a feather. The procedure turned out to be that feather. Daniel helped him enroll in hospice care, and Rick died peacefully in his sleep, in his own home, nine months later.

"House of Cards" describes a state of health as precarious as a structure built of playing cards, and it is common in people in their nineties or in the mid to later stages of dementia. When they take a "great fall," it's unlikely that all the king's horses and all the king's men will ever put them back together again. Counterintuitive as it seems, *protection from* inappropriate forms of medicine can now be at least as important as *access to* the care that helps most—the majority of which will be gentle and, if possible, delivered at home. Good medical care now includes finding a physician house call service, shifting to a focus on comfort, upgrading advance directives, thinking through a pathway to a peaceful death, and doing everything possible to reduce the risk of a traumatic hospital stay or emergency room visit. The most realistic goal now may simply be this: to not make a bad situation worse.

This can be a confusing shift to navigate. The hope of improvement from a last-ditch medical technology is tantalizing. Ever since Eli Whitney invented the cotton gin, our culture has nourished the illusion that technological advances will soon usher in a utopia. But in the words of grief counselor Meghan Devine, "Some things in life cannot be fixed. They can only be carried."

Most people in the House of Cards have "the dwindles" or are on a looping or stair step trajectory of final decline. About a quarter of Americans become frail in their seventies. By the age of eighty-one, about 40 percent of us are frail. Very fit and resilient people, about a quarter of the aging population, will reach the end of their lives having spent only a few weeks or months being frail.

RECOGNIZING FRAILTY

It's important to recognize frailty as a distinct health stage, because medical approaches that helped earlier can now harm. Now is the time to eliminate medical risks, to lower one's expectations of medicine, and to get clear on what "living well" means as life is slowly winding down. If you, or someone you care for, is still on the conveyor belt of fragmented, crisis-focused medical care, with a focus on prolonging life rather than preserving function and relieving suffering, it's wise to find a way off.

Frail people in coordinated health systems tend to do better than those outside them. When an array of individual specialists try to fix the multiple problems of frailty, they often fail to notice the overarching concerns of many families and patients. Most frail people want to reduce burdens on their caregivers. They need practical support, like daycare programs, housekeeping, or Meals on Wheels, and they fear having to move into a nursing home. Doctors' appointments and unnecessary trips to the emergency room exhaust them.

But people rarely talk to their doctors about these concerns. Somehow they don't seem "medical" enough. Within the hypnotic purview of the doctor's office there's often an assumption that improving scores on tests and postponing death is everyone's number one goal. But it may be more realistic—and important— to enjoy the moment, to love and be loved, to accept help, and to plan for a good death, even though it may be a year or two away. Unless you discuss your concerns openly, you and your doctor may not be on the same page. So speak up. Continue to bring up what matters most to you (or to the person you care for) even if it's mundane and modest, like continuing to live at home, to walk, to play music, or to enjoy your grandchildren.

AVOIDING THE HOSPITAL

In an all-too-common scenario, a frail person faints, falls, or has a minor medical problem that in an earlier era would have simply been called a "spell" and overlooked or handled by a family doctor who came to the house. Today, that overly busy and underpaid medical point person, now known bureaucratically as your "primary care provider," may not even squeeze in a same-day appointment or have a nurse return your phone call. In assisted living residences without house call services, state regulations usually require immediate medical attention after any "medical event." This often means a call to 911 after even a minor fall.

The only recourse, especially after hours or on weekends, is likely to be the emergency room, where the frail elderly often sit for hours while doctors attend first to those with life-threatening infections, heart attacks, and injuries. In the cruel slang of the hospital, frustrated doctors in training may covertly refer to them as "frequent flyers." After numerous tests, the frail elder goes home, often with the original problem unresolved, or is admitted for a brief hospital stay, followed by three weeks in an unfamiliar nursing home. For the still vigorous, a nursing home stay for physical rehabilitation can restore function. But for the severely frail, especially the demented, the stress and disorientation often results in a major step down in functioning. This cycle repeats over and over, exhausting caregivers, medical and institutional staff, and patients alike. Dr. Eileen Callahan of Mount Sinai hospital in Manhattan says, "What we try to do as geriatricians is keep patients out of the hospital at all costs. It's often a life-changing event."

Frail people should go to the emergency room only for things the ER handles well: intractable pain requiring intravenous painkillers; a broken bone or a wound that requires stitches; uncontrolled bleeding; a fever of over 104; a rampant infection requiring intravenous antibiotics; or symptoms of a stroke that requires immediate treatment with clot-busting medication. If someone is already too weak to withstand surgery, there's no need to put them through stressful diagnostic tests like CAT scans that won't change the course of treatment.

If a frail person has a minor fall and can't be gotten up, consider skipping 911 and instead calling the business line of the local fire department and asking for their "Lift and Assist" service. Be clear that this is a "nonemergency lift" (use exactly that language) and say that you just want two burly firefighters, not paramedics, to show up at the house and help the frail person up. Another option, albeit riskier, is to call 911 and again emphasize that this is a "nonemergency lift." Once paramedics arrive in their ambulance, however, they may try quite forcefully to persuade the elder to go to the hospital.

Don't feel you *must* go. Fainting and falling by themselves are not emergencies: they're often a fact of life at this health stage. A fall can result from getting up from a chair too fast, eating or drinking too little, getting overheated, picking up a urinary tract infection, having a slow heartbeat, having a bad reaction to an antidepressant like Prozac, or taking too much medication to lower blood pressure or blood sugar. None of these are best treated in an emergency room. Consider drinking water, resting, and setting up an outpatient appointment at an urgent care center or with a primary care physician. (In a coordinated HMO, you may be able to call a twenty-four-hour advice nurse or go to its urgent care department.) Bring in all pill bottles, including supplements, for a medication review. You can then explore options in a calmer atmosphere.

The same cautionary principles apply to surgery. Before agreeing to any invasive procedure, I recommend you assess where you stand (or someone you're responsible for stands) in relation to the three elements critical to a decent recovery:

- *Energy.* If it takes all available energy just to get through the day, little surplus will be left for healing. According to geriatrics specialist Eric Widera, MD, those who cannot walk half a mile under their own power are at high risk of returning from surgery with worsened disabilities.
- *Muscle mass.* Even a few days in a hospital bed leads to muscle wasting. People too weak to rise easily from a chair may never recover the ability to stand up on their own.
- *Acuity.* If a simple "mini mental status exam" shows mild or moderate dementia, you are at serious risk of becoming confused and having hallucinations in the hospital, a destructive condition called "hospital delirium." Delirium was once thought to be passing, but many older people who suffer it never recover critical mental and physical function. Three-quarters end up in nursing homes, and 35 to 40 percent die within a year.

If you score badly on these red flags, but simply must go, family and friends should stand guard against disorientation, exhaustion, and medication errors. Bring hearing aids and eyeglasses, as they reduce confusion and helplessness. Ear plugs and eye masks will help you sleep, and so will asking the charge nurse or an attending physician for a medical order prohibiting anyone from awakening you at night to take vital signs. Ask friends to bring in healthy take-out food or favorite dishes from home and share a meal. Check all medications given—overdoses and mix-ups are common—and ask medical staff courteously to wash their hands before touching you, to reduce infection risk. You may feel more like yourself if you wear your own pajamas and post family photographs where you can see them. It's best to keep hospital stays brief, and to get home as soon as possible. If you think you'd do better at home, you can leave "against medical advice" (AMA) as do about fifty thousand older people a year. Some sign hospital paperwork acknowledging the risks, and others simply get out.

FINDING ALLIES IN HOUSE CALL PROGRAMS

The dangers of hospitalization can be beautifully avoided by returning to an ancient medical practice, standard from the days of Hippocrates to mid-twentieth-century America: the physician (or nurse) house call. These programs are being revived: the gold standard here is the Veterans Administration's well-regarded Home Based Primary Care Program (HBPC), which cares for tens of thousands of seriously ill veterans in their own homes. Currently available only to the sickest 5 percent of vets, it has the highest satisfaction rating of any VA program . . . and long waiting lists. People who get in sometimes say they feel as if they've won the lottery.

A nurse case manager makes sure everyone stays on the same page and nips budding health problems before they bloom into crises. Doctors and nurses make house calls, and so do social workers, occupational and physical therapists, and technicians who do X-rays on the spot and draw blood for diagnostic tests. Some Medicare Advantage programs and other all-under-one-roof health systems offer similar, but less extensive programs (like Aspire, offered in many parts of the South and Midwest). These programs are sometimes called "pre-hospice," "serious illness management," or "home-based palliative care," so it helps to ask for them under these terms.

If none is available, I recommend finding a private physician who makes house calls, or adding on a free-standing program, like the late lamented DASH (Doctors Assisting Seniors at Home), program in Santa Barbara, California, which provided nurse house calls under a physician's direction from 2012 to 2018. It reduced emergency room visits in its members by an average of 40 percent. Retired nurse Katina Etsell, for instance, was caring for both her parents, who were in their nineties. One relied on a walker, the other on a wheelchair. Their health problems were usually too pressing to wait for days for a regular doctor's appointment, but rarely serious enough to warrant hours in the ER.

"We'd get a doctor's appointment for days or a week down the line, when we wanted to deal with it right then," said Katina, who is in her sixties. "And getting them to the office required transferring them from wheelchairs and walkers into the car. I could do it, but it was just so hard for me."

For ninety dollars a month, Katina enrolled both parents in DASH. The service was a supplement—the couple kept their personal doctors. But when they had urgent problems, especially after hours and on Saturdays, Katina called DASH. A visiting nurse would usually arrive at the house within twenty-four hours. Conferring by phone with a supervising doctor, the nurse could run blood or urine tests on the spot.

When problems couldn't be resolved at home, the DASH nurse and her supervising doctor referred the couple to their personal physicians. When Katina's late father developed a boil on his head caused by the potentially deadly antibiotic-resistant bacterium MRSA, for instance, the DASH nurse sent him to his doctor, who lanced the boil in an office visit and put him on a powerful antibiotic. When that drug provoked gastrointestinal bleeding, Katina called the DASH nurse, and she suggested trying Prilosec before taking him to the ER. Luckily, the bleeding responded promptly to the over-the-counter drug. In the course of four years, Katina figures, DASH saved her parents nearly a dozen visits to doctors' offices and emergency rooms.

Each of DASH's nurses carried a briefcase containing thirty commonly prescribed drugs. They could hand out a two-day supply and arrange for a full prescription to be called in by a DASH doctor to a local pharmacy.

DASH also saw people who lived in nursing homes and assisted living residences—a godsend for residents who'd had a minor fall and would plead not to be bundled off to the ER. It was free to people of any age on Medicaid in Santa Barbara. Single people on Medicare paid sixty dollars a month, and couples, ninety.

Even though programs like DASH save insurers hundreds of thousands of dollars by reducing ambulance rides and ER visits that can easily top $10,000 per incident, they're poorly reimbursed by insurance, and therefore scarce. DASH, unfortunately, folded in 2018. But similar programs still exist, all across the country, and they're worth seeking out.

Many are financially supported by a pilot Medicare program, folded within the Affordable Care Act, called "Independence At Home." (It is one of many small, imaginative Medicare initiatives that should be expanded to cover everyone who needs them.) Among them are Doctors on Call in Brooklyn, New York; the Visiting Physicians Association in Flint, Michigan; House Call Providers of Portland, Oregon; and others listed on page 241. You can find others, such as the excellent House Call Program at the

University of California at San Francisco (UCSF) within medical school geriatrics departments, which train young doctors.

Even if you must pay out-of-pocket, try to find a house call or visiting nurse program if you can afford it. Many private house call doctors are listed by zip code on the websites of the American Academy of Home Care Medicine and the Visiting Physicians Association. If you can't find one, give yourself credit for trying: these needed services are few and far between.

UPGRADING ADVANCE DIRECTIVES

To reduce the chances of putting yourself (or an elder whom you care for) through one or more grueling and futile end-of-life medical experiences, I suggest upgrading the advance directive to a more detailed Physician's Order for Life-Sustaining Treatment, or POLST. (In some states, this is called a Medical Order for Life-Sustaining Treatment, or MOLST.) A portable one-page document printed on bright pink paper, a POLST is filled out by a doctor, in consultation with the patient or the health care advocate. Because they are official "doctors' orders," they carry much more weight within health systems than do advance directives, which are "only" signed by the patient.

The POLST or MOLST gives you a chance to acknowledge that many once-desired medical interventions are now unwanted. Honored in most states, they are revolutionary because they break down institutional silos and are recognized by nursing home staff, emergency medical personnel, and hospitals alike. Many family caregivers and nurses say that POLSTs are frequently lost or misfiled, so keep multiple backups, all copied on bright pink paper.

Most POLSTs and MOLSTs list three options:

- *Comfort Measures Only*, which allows painkillers but forbids antibiotics, CPR, intravenous fluids, and ambulance trips to the hospital.

- *Limited Treatment*, which permits antibiotics and IV fluids, but forbids aggressive measures like CPR or intubation, and may or may not permit transport to a hospital, depending on which boxes are checked.
- *Full Treatment*, which means doing everything possible to prolong life: resuscitations, tests, medications, transport to a hospital, placement on a ventilator, and admission to intensive care.

Asking a doctor to sign a POLST does not automatically mean welcoming death with open arms. It's not an invitation for medical neglect or a way of saying "do not treat me." Many people, for instance, are fine with antibiotics and intravenous fluids, but not with more invasive treatments. Your doctors are not your moral arbiters—nor are your relatives. There are no wrong answers. Your choices will reflect your deepest sense of what is right *for you*. (When people have dementia, their medical advocates should fill out POLSTs on their behalf, as I will discuss later in this chapter.)

POLSTs usually include a separate line for a do-not-resuscitate order (DNR), sometimes called an "allow natural death" (AND) order. This is a mercy, because CPR for the frail is brutal and usually ineffective. Fewer than 8 percent of people over age seventy resuscitated outside a hospital ever return to independent living. Almost all suffer pain and trauma during an attempted resuscitation, which includes shocking the heart with an electric defibrillator and forcefully pushing on the chest, often breaking brittle ribs. Some die within hours, days, or weeks of one or more attempted resuscitations, while others survive with permanent brain damage. Emergency room staff often suffer "moral distress" when they feel torn between allowing a gentle natural death, and adhering to the hospital's protocols, which in the absence of a POLST usually require "doing everything" to prevent death, no matter how futile and painful.

A doctor can also write up a DNR as a freestanding medical order, but depending on regulations that differ state by state, paper DNRs are not always honored by paramedics who respond to 911 calls. (A notable exception is Oregon, which trains all its paramedics to immediately recognize and honor POLSTs and DNRs.) This has led some ICU nurses to get chest tattoos reading "no code" or "do not resuscitate." But medical staff sometimes ignore even these bold inked messages if they're not backed up by official paperwork!

The only DNR symbol recognized in every state is a metal bracelet, similar to an allergy alert, obtainable from the Medic Alert Foundation with a doctor's order. (Many states issue plastic bracelets valid only in their state.) Keep in mind that if a frail person arrives at an emergency room in extremis, without an advance directive or a vigilant family member, all systems will usually spring into action to prevent death.

Keep the POLST and DNR forms on the door of the refrigerator, along with the document naming a health care decision maker. Put laminated copies in the trunk or glove compartment of the cars of anyone who might drive the frail person to the hospital. As ever, it's crucial that all caregivers understand what the patient wants (and doesn't want) and are willing to abide by it. Prior discussions with family members, confirmed in a written POLST, have helped many people in a crisis.

COPING WITH DEMENTIA

Dementia was once conceived of as one of many forms of mental impairment. But doctors, led by the pioneering dementia specialist Susan Mitchell of Harvard University, are increasingly describing it as a terminal illness, albeit one that moves at a glacial pace. It affects not just the brain but the entire nervous system. In its end stages, sufferers not only lose the ability to recognize loved ones but forget how to chew, swallow, walk, and sit up. Being bedbound ushers in a cascade of problems, often including a fatal pneumonia or a urinary tract infection. Dementia sufferers can benefit from palliative care, and eventually hospice, just as much as people with any other fatal illness. But few get it.

Because medical technologies can now prolong the lives of people with dementia almost indefinitely, their caregivers face moral dilemmas unknown to earlier generations and unaddressed by Hippocrates. At a time when a daughter, son, or spouse may be overwhelmed with caregiving, or may want to grieve and simply be present, he or she may be called upon to decide when to stop medically prolonging a life that has become filled with suffering.

Unfortunately, few caregivers have the benefit of advance directives that directly address dementia, and our demented relatives usually can no longer express their wishes. In the absence of clear guidance, relatives often opt to allow more uncomfortable, life-prolonging treatments than they might choose for themselves. Nothing can make this easy, but I hope the following suggestions will help.

If you are the health care agent, I recommend you start by asking for a sketch of the trajectory of the illness, where your loved one is on the trajectory, and what you can expect in the future. In light of this information, I suggest the following exercise. Imagine that the old, fully functioning "self" of the person you love, by some miracle, could return to you in full mental and physical health for fifteen minutes. Lay the situation before them, and listen to what they would say. I did this when my mother asked me to help her get my father's pacemaker deactivated. I vividly imagined him sitting at the kitchen table, and shaking his head in horror at what his life had become. It gave me the strength to support my mother and to ask my father's doctors to deactivate the device.

You might also get clues from your loved one's behavior, especially if they are miserable, agitated, tied down, or drugged. Ask yourself what you would want if you were in their shoes, and what course of action will leave you with the fewest regrets.

There is no consensus in our society, religiously or medically, on the moral path forward. This is uncharted territory. Orthodox Judaism prohibits even removing a pillow from beneath a dying man's head if it will hasten death by a minute. The Catholic Church has repeatedly stated that its followers do not have to submit to "extraordinary measures" (like ventilators) to prolong life, but adds that our lives belong to God, not to ourselves, and should be lived for His glory. Some doctors push for feeding tubes, saying things like "nobody starves to death on my watch," while other doctors view prescribing medications to hasten a difficult death as an act of compassion. Given this wide range of moral stances, you must delve into your own beliefs and make decisions on behalf of people whom you love deeply, know well, and are responsible for. You may find yourself challenging medical protocols or facing the moral judgments of others. If so, I hope you find comfort, as I do, in the words of the philosopher Zygmunt Bauman. "Uncertainty is not a temporary nuisance which can be chased away through learning the rules, or surrendering to expert advice or just doing what others do. Instead it is a permanent condition of life. . . . To be responsible does not mean to follow the rules. It may often require us to disregard the rules or to act in ways the rules do not warrant."

I personally believe that death is part of God's (or Nature's) plan, and that a loving God never intended to force people to suffer at the hands of advanced technologies that cannot restore them. Yes, the Bible recounts miraculous healings, but its miracles are grounded in faith, not in man-made inventions with a potential for both good and evil. It's hard to morally justify putting people through regimens that cause them suffering when they can neither understand the purpose of the pain inflicted, nor meaningfully assent to it. We must normalize saying "no": depriving a demented person of a natural death may seem loving, but it is rarely kind. The suffering of caregivers also deserves moral weight. If your doctor is not on the same page, find another more attuned to your values.

The double-edged medical technologies you are most likely to confront are: CPR, dialysis, ventilators, implanted cardiac defibrillators, pacemakers, feeding tubes, intravenous lines for drugs and saline solutions, and antibiotics. All delay death, often painfully, without restoring well-being. Antibiotics can deprive someone of the blessing of a relatively gentle death from pneumonia, once called "the old man's friend." Artificial hydration can draw out dying for weeks. Many patients with feeding tubes are drugged or tied down to prevent them from pulling them out. For more detailed guidance, I highly recommend the Alzheimer's Association's free pamphlet "End of Life Decisions," and the book *Hard Choices for Loving People*, written by hospice chaplain Hank Dunn.

Sometimes a family advocate must become a warrior. That was the case for Karen Randall, a veterinarian in Washington, D.C., when her father, Ed Walski, entered the House of Cards. Ed was a widower in his early eighties who'd spent his working life at IBM, repairing mainframes in the days when computers took up entire rooms and then moving into management. He had dementia and Parkinson's disease.

In the last year of his life, staff at Ed's assisted living complex sent him to the hospital nine times—sometimes because he'd fallen; often because he was agitated and screaming, perhaps due to untreated pain; and sometimes because he had a urinary tract infection or pneumonia. The first few times, Karen rushed to meet the ambulance at the hospital and did what she assumed was the loving, caring thing. She insisted doctors pull out all the stops, run every possible test, and as she put it, "find out what was causing his bizarre changes in behavior and fix it." Her father repeatedly had his blood drawn and his urine analyzed, followed by CAT scans, MRIs, X-rays, and echocardiograms. "I really needed answers," she remembers. "I wanted my dad back."

The tests were often inconclusive, and after three days in the hospital and sometimes treatment with antibiotics, Ed would go to a nursing home for three weeks of rehabilitation. "I'd say, okay, we got him through this and now he's going to get rehab and be back where he was," Karen said. "But he never came back. It was a stair step down to the basement."

Karen realized that "these hospitalizations weren't improving anybody's quality of life," she said. "The illnesses were attempting to take him, and we just wouldn't let them. My father never smiled. His life had gotten miserable. I was watching him growing more and more angry and frustrated and incapable. But nobody was offering us any alternative."

She shifted her focus from *cure* to *comfort*. She asked his assisted living residence not to send him to the emergency room, and tried to get him enrolled in hospice. But the residence wouldn't budge from their standard protocols, and the hospice turned him down: neither Parkinson's nor the early stages of dementia are hospice-qualifying diagnoses.

During his final ER visit, after yet another fall, doctors asked Karen to authorize a swallowing test. The staff was worried that his pneumonias were being caused by inhaling tiny bits of food because of poor swallowing. The test results could pave the way for inserting a feeding tube.

Karen said no. If she wasn't going to authorize the tube, she saw no reason to allow the test. Years earlier, her father had signed a POLST document and appointed her as his health care advocate. "I was able to flash back to him saying, 'Hell no! I don't want any feeding tubes!'" she said. "That almost made it easy." But not too easy. Three times in one day, Karen was asked—by a nurse, a social worker, and a nursing supervisor—whether she understood that without a feeding tube, her father might develop a pneumonia that could kill him. She stuck to her refusal. When her father was discharged, she moved him to a smaller assisted living complex, this one run by an RN who agreed to do her best to keep Ed out of the hospital. He died in the new place three weeks later, of yet another pneumonia. Karen was able to get him qualified for hospice only three days before he died, on the basis of a diagnosis of Lewy body dementia, which *is* a hospice qualifying diagnosis. After months of falling through the cracks in the system, Ed's final days were peaceful.

"When you start out, you want to do the best for them, and it takes a while to figure out where things are going," Karen said. "At the end, when I was making the big decisions and everybody was questioning me, I was really struggling. I expected to be left with a lot of questions. But after he died, everything became clear to me. I was proud of the way I had helped him leave this world. It didn't feel right at the time, but it sure did in hindsight."

SHIFTING TO COMFORT CARE

Consider asking doctors to switch to "comfort care measures only." The phrase "comfort care" helps everyone involved feel more comfortable—not only the gravely ill, but their family members, medical teams, and nursing home staff. Simply stating what you *don't want* can provoke resistance and make some staff members feel they are being asked to abandon a patient. Asking for what you *do want* provides them with alternative ways to express their caring, and is an achievable goal. It is almost always possible to reduce someone's suffering.

Comfort care is what it sounds like: saying *yes* to medical attention that keeps a person comfortable and *no* to any treatment that causes pain or distress. This simple little phrase is widely used but not explicitly defined in the medical world. Practically speaking, it means gentle, noninvasive care for people who aren't officially on the hospice benefit and therefore can't be seen or billed by a hospice team. Many doctors who have spent their careers devoted to people with dementia believe that "comfort measures only" ought to be the standard of care for their patients.

It is what I want if I develop dementia. Here is the letter I've written, as an amendment to my advance directive, to guide my medical advocates. It contains a thorough description of my conception of comfort care.

Dear Medical Advocate;

If you're reading this because I can't make my own medical decisions due to dementia, please understand I don't wish to prolong my living or dying, even if I seem relatively happy and content. As a human being who currently has the moral and intellectual capacity to make my own decisions, I want you to know that I care about the emotional, financial, and practical burdens that dementia and similar illnesses place on those who love me. Once I am demented, I may become oblivious to such concerns. So please let my wishes as stated below guide you.

- I wish to remove all barriers to a natural, peaceful, and timely death.

- Please ask my medical team to provide Comfort Care Only.

- Try to qualify me for hospice.

- I do not wish any attempt at resuscitation. Ask my doctor to sign a do-not-resuscitate order and order me a do-not-resuscitate bracelet from the Medic Alert Foundation.

- Ask my medical team to allow natural death. Do not authorize any medical procedure that might prolong or delay my death.

- Do not transport me to a hospital. I prefer to die in the place that has become my home.

- Do not intubate me or give me intravenous fluids. I do not want treatments that may prolong or increase my suffering.

- Do not treat my infections with antibiotics, give me painkillers instead.

- Ask my doctor to deactivate all medical devices, such as defibrillators, that may delay death and cause pain.

- Ask my doctor to deactivate any medical device that might delay death, even those, such as pacemakers, that may improve my comfort.

- If I'm eating, let me eat what I want, and don't put me on "thickened liquids," even if this increases my risk of pneumonia.

- Do not force or coax me to eat.

- Do not authorize a feeding tube for me, even on a trial basis. If one is inserted, please ask for its immediate removal.

- Ask to stop, and do not give permission to start, dialysis.

- Do not agree to any tests whose results would be meaningless, given my desire to avoid treatments that might be burdensome, agitating, painful, or prolonging of my life or death.

- Do not give me a flu or other vaccine that might delay my death, unless required to protect others.

- Do keep me out of physical pain, with opioids if necessary.

- Ask my doctor to fill out the medical orders known as POLST (Physician Orders for Life-Sustaining Treatment) or MOLST (Medical Orders for Life-Sustaining Treatment) to confirm the wishes I've expressed here.

- If I must be institutionalized, please do your best to find a place with art workshops and access to nature, if I can still enjoy them.

ENJOYING YOUR RED VELVET CAKE

Most people in the House of Cards stage have two years or less to live. There is little future to sacrifice for. This is a turning point: from fighting to stay functional to accepting decline, savoring the brief time left, and looking forward to preparing for a peaceful death. Enjoy the day.

If you want to (or a frail person you care for wants to) eat bacon and ice cream, indulge. Good eating habits pay off over decades, not months. Exercise and physical therapy can still help maintain function, but some people with dwindling energy and multiple ailments simply refuse it. If you're a caregiver, it's time to stop nagging and let go.

Many geriatrics specialists recommend lightening up on tight control of cholesterol, blood pressure, and blood sugar. Blood pressure medications can increase the risk of falls. Severe diabetic complications take years to develop and many doctors take a more relaxed attitude toward moderately elevated blood sugar in frail elderly patients. Go along with them. For people with limited pleasures, enjoying favorite foods may be more important than reducing, infinitesimally, their time on earth. If you're hyper-focused on seeking aggressive medical care for a declining loved one, ask yourself whether anxiety about impending loss is skewing your judgment. Many people in the House of Cards feel better when their doctors reduce other medications and focus more closely on managing pain.

Parse medical appointments carefully, and ponder which are effective. I think it's worthwhile to keep nurturing a good ongoing relationship with a geriatrician or personal doctor, to have a yearly medication review, to update advance directives with each change in health, and to have a specialist or nurse case manager carefully manage chronic problems like congestive heart failure. But if you are going to a specialist's office merely to monitor and document a condition (like dementia) for which no good treatments exist, consider cutting back, unless you need the evidence to qualify for hospice or another benefit. *You* decide how you want to spend your days, and the energy of your caregivers. By the same token, have a frank discussion with a doctor about getting a medical order to deactivate an internal cardiac defibrillator, if it hasn't been done already. Its shocks are painful, will rarely prolong life by more than a few months, and can interfere with a peaceful death. In all things, make sure that medical treatment improves how you feel or function, and doesn't burden you or waste your precious time.

Dietrich Mayer is six feet four and solidly built, a car mechanic who grew up in Queens Village, New York. When his mother, Betty, was widowed in her sixties, Dietrich and his wife bought a bigger house farther out on Long Island, with a separate apartment for Betty. She did well throughout her seventies and eighties, entertaining her grandchildren, knitting afghans for her nephews and nieces, walking to the local grocery store to shop, and doing her own laundry and cooking.

In her early nineties, Betty fell twice on her way home—once carrying a big bottle of bleach, and another time lugging a sack of potatoes. She began having brief mental blank spots when she seemed to lose consciousness for a couple of minutes, and then "come back," apparently fine. Commonly called "TIAs" (transient ischemic attacks) these mini-strokes are temporary blockages of blood flow in the brain and usually resolve quickly. But the micro-damage can add up, promoting forgetfulness.

One autumn day, Dietrich took his mother to a big family event, an eightieth birthday party honoring his mother-in-law, held in a hotel ballroom. Betty was among the guests singing "Happy Birthday" and had just been handed a slice of red velvet cake when she started mumbling and shaking, until she lost consciousness. When she didn't revive after a minute or two, Dietrich and his brother-in-law, a police officer, picked up Betty's chair with her in it and carried her to the hotel entrance. Paramedics arrived within minutes. By then, Betty was awake and insisting she didn't want to go to the hospital. But at the urging of his brother-in-law, Dietrich convinced her to do so, and followed her ambulance in his car.

At the hospital, doctors ran tests, all inconclusive. Betty kept saying she just wanted to return to the party.

A doctor entered the room. She told Dietrich that the hospital planned to keep Betty overnight, to run more tests and see if she needed a pacemaker. Dietrich drew himself up to his considerable height. "That ain't friggin' going to happen," he said. "My mother needs to come home. All she wants to do is finish her cake."

The doctor said that Dietrich would have to first sign paper-work acknowledging that he was taking his mother away "against medical advice." Dietrich did so. The doctor shut the door, moved close to Dietrich, and said under her breath, "I can't tell you this officially, but they do so much better when you just take them home."

Over the next five years, this pattern was repeated during multiple hospital visits, until Betty entered a nursing home. At the suggestion of its director, Dietrich obtained a MOLST, signed by Betty's doctor, indicating that she was not to be transported to the hospital for any reason. She died peacefully at the nursing home, at the age of ninety-seven, in her own bed.

Now get back to the party and enjoy your red velvet cake.

Ways to Prepare:

- Recognize advanced frailty and protect yourself, or someone you love, from medical overtreatment.
- Avoid the emergency room and the hospital. Find home-based medical care if you can. Consider a shift to comfort care.
- Get a POLST or MOLST signed by a doctor and consider a do-not-resuscitate (DNR) or allow natural death (AND) order. Get a physician's order to deactivate an implanted defibrillator. POLST and MOLST forms for each state are available at POLST Paradigm (Polst.org).
- Consider halting dialysis.
- Relax dietary and other restrictions. Enjoy the time that remains.

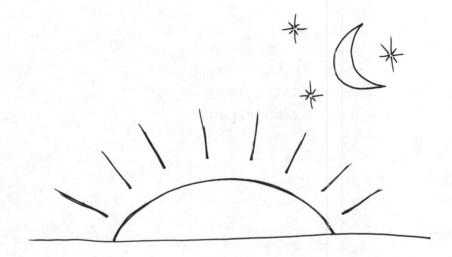

CHAPTER 6

Preparing for a Good Death

Making Good Use of the Time You Have Left
Finding Allies in Hospice • Next Steps
Settling Your Affairs • Choosing the Time of Death
Loving, Thanking, and Forgiving • Getting Help from Your Tribe

Awakened

In advanced age, my health worsening,
I woke up in the middle of the night
and experienced a feeling of happiness
so intense and perfect that in all my life
I had only felt its premonition.
And there was no reason for it.
It didn't obliterate consciousness;
the past, which I carried, was there,
together with my grief.
And it was suddenly included,
was a necessary part of the whole.
As if a voice were repeating:
"You can stop worrying now;
everything happened just as it had to.
You did what was assigned to you,
and you are not required anymore
to think of what happened long ago."
The peace I felt was a closing of accounts
and was connected with the thought of death.
The happiness on this side was
like an announcement of the other side.
I realized that this was an undeserved gift
and I could not grasp by what grace
it was bestowed on me.

—CZESLAW MILOSZ, written not long before
his death at the age of ninety-three

You may find this chapter helpful if your death is six months to a year away. It is directed toward those still making their own medical decisions, and to the people who will care for them. You are in this health stage if you recognize yourself in some of the following statements:

- If asked, your doctors would say that they wouldn't be surprised if you died within a year.
- You've lost 10 percent or more of your body weight in the past six months.
- You have a terminal diagnosis and doctors say your illness is "advanced" or is reaching its "end stages."
- Cancer has returned after two or more rounds of treatment, you have decided not to undergo more, or a doctor has said "there's nothing more we can do for you."
- A friend, family member, or doctor has suggested hospice.
- You've refused dialysis, a defibrillator, or other life-prolonging technology. Alternatively, you want to stop some forms of treatment.
- You say or think things like "Why am I still alive?" "No more hospitals," or "I'm ready for God to take me."
- You feel life is no longer worth living. This is a highly individual judgment: some people enjoy life with health conditions that others can't abide.
- If you haven't already, you feel the urge to reconcile old conflicts, forgive people who've hurt you, and otherwise make peace.
- If you haven't already, you deepen your interest in spiritual questions, reconnect with your old religious tradition, or explore a new path.
- If you haven't done so earlier, you begin to make funeral plans, give away clothes, or throw out old papers so you don't leave a mess for your kids.

MAKING GOOD USE OF THE TIME YOU HAVE LEFT

When Mary Jane Denzer was diagnosed with pancreatic cancer, her first reaction was to fight it. She was eighty-two and full of life. Aside from being slightly nauseous after eating a meal, she felt completely healthy. She ran her own dress shop in White Plains, New York, and walked several long blocks to work every day, usually in high-heeled boots. She spent her days scurrying between clothes racks and dressing rooms filled with customers. She loved her life, her four adult children, her dog, and her grandchildren. Twice a year she went to Europe to see the designer shows and order new clothes for her store. She wasn't ready for any of it to end.

Soon after her diagnosis, she saw an oncologist at Manhattan's Memorial Sloan-Kettering, one of the nation's preeminent cancer research and treatment centers. The doctor was honest. Surgery wasn't an option. The tumor, originating in Mary Jane's pancreas, had wrapped around a huge artery branching from her aorta, the body's largest blood vessel. Trying to surgically remove the tumor, the oncologist said, might rupture the artery, cause uncontrollable bleeding, and kill her.

That didn't mean that Sloan-Kettering had nothing for her. The oncologist offered her three courses of treatment. The harshest chemotherapy might give Mary Jane more time, or it might kill her quicker than her cancer. A less grueling chemo might temporarily keep death at bay, but it would make her hair fall out. The mildest chemo might preserve her hair, but it would give her no more than an extra month. No matter what she chose, the oncologist said, Mary Jane was unlikely to live more than six months.

The oncologist raised another possibility: hospice.

Mary Jane said no. She wanted to "fight." She opted for the mildest chemo.

For three weeks straight, she went to a beautifully appointed suburban branch of the cancer center and lay down in a recliner while the drug was infused into her veins. When given to patients with fatal cancers, this approach is sometimes called "palliative chemotherapy."

The stated goal of palliative chemotherapy is to relieve suffering and improve the quality of the patient's remaining life, not to root out the disease, which doctors know is impossible. But the phrase makes some palliative care doctors bristle, because it can be a contradiction in terms. In the wrong circumstances, palliative chemo can be anything but palliative. Instead of soothing symptoms, it can make people feel sicker, and make their deaths more difficult, without increasing their survival times at all.

Mary Jane didn't know this. And even though nobody at the cancer center misled her, who can blame her? The center where she was being treated was one of the best known in the nation. Its recent million-dollar advertising campaign had featured full-page ads in national magazines showing healthy-looking, apparently victorious patients holding up signs saying things like "Cancer, NICE TRY."

After three weeks of chemotherapy, some of Mary Jane's hair fell out. Her lungs filled with fluid. She had trouble breathing. She was admitted to a hospital near her home, where she picked up *Clostridium difficile,* a devastating, antibiotic-resistant gut infection. Rampant in American hospitals, *C. diff* is spread by the overuse of antibiotics and the careless washing of bedding, equipment, and doctors' and nurses' hands. It causes excruciating and sometimes fatal diarrhea, especially in the elderly and in those whose immune systems are already compromised by illness or chemotherapy.

By the time Mary Jane left the hospital, the triple blow of cancer, chemotherapy, and *C. diff* had almost killed her. She weighed a hundred pounds and looked skeletal. She was, as she told me, "knocked for a loop." Deciding she was on the brink of death, Mary Jane told her doctor to stop chemo. "It was only going to give me another month, and it made me so much sicker it wasn't worth it," she said matter-of-factly. "It's worth it if you're going to get better. But it's not worth it if you're not."

One of her four children, her daughter Cathryn Ramin, helped Mary Jane enroll in a local hospice program. Money was not a problem, and the family made arrangements for a private agency to provide hands-on caregiving. Everyone braced for what they thought would be the quick arrival of the inevitable. That wasn't the expectation of Kelly, the lead hospice nurse.

In Kelly's opinion, Mary Jane's life wasn't over just because she had stopped fighting death. Once the side effects of the chemo and *C. diff* receded and Mary Jane's pain was controlled with small doses of morphine, she returned, with Kelly's encouragement, to doing what she loved. That meant seeing her friends, children, and grandchildren; pampering her dog; buying clothes for herself and her store; and continuing to walk to work and run her dress shop— all while "on hospice."

"My first reaction was, oh my gosh, I really am dying," Mary Jane told me seven months after she enrolled in hospice. "But you're not really dying yet. You can make good use of the time you have left. You just don't know how long it's going to be."

Several times a week, her daughter Cathryn would take the train from New York City to join her mother for dinner in White Plains. "I'd arrive around six o'clock," Cathryn said. "A lot of times the apartment was dead dark, nobody was there, and nothing had been planned for dinner. I'd come up to visit the sick and dying, and the supposedly 'sick and dying' was still at work!"

Some people think hospices provide little medical care beyond morphine in the final hours of life. That wasn't the case for

Mary Jane. It's true that when she shifted to hospice, she had to say goodbye to her doctors at the cancer center and hand over all her medical care to the hospice team. It's also true that her tumors kept growing until they distended her stomach. Her pain increased, along with the morphine doses she used to manage it.

But she was healthier and happier, and she probably lived longer than she would have if she'd continued with so-called palliative chemotherapy, or doubled down on a harsher medical assault, the one that many stage four cancer patients and their doctors wage against death until a few weeks before the end.

Hospice did not mean medical neglect. When her tumors interfered with her pancreas's ability to regulate her blood sugar, a hospice nurse put her on a stringent diet to manage her resulting diabetes, and she felt better. When the tumors spread to her liver, a hospice doctor sent her to the hospital, where stents were inserted to open her blocked bile ducts and relieve her jaundice. When her abdomen swelled with fluids and pressed on her lungs, causing breathlessness, she returned to the hospital, again as an outpatient, to have the fluid drained. She breathed more easily. As her pain increased, she graduated from morphine drops placed under the tongue to higher-dose tablets and finally to morphine delivered by intravenous pump. The hospice's focus on the quality of her life had a strange side effect: it extended it.

Outfoxing all predictions, Mary Jane lived for a full year after engaging hospice. She had the time, comfort, freedom from pain, and mental clarity to arrange a reconciliatory lunch with an estranged former sister-in-law. She wrote her daughter Cathryn a beautiful letter thanking her for her love and caregiving. She bought expensive new boots even though she didn't have time to wear them out. She kept going to work, although at increasingly reduced hours, until six weeks before her death. She died in her own home, with her family around her.

Preparing for death—practically, emotionally, and spiritually—tends to intensify when dying is between six months and a year away. Some people arrive at this crossroads unwillingly, when a doctor tells them that further treatment won't buy them more time. Others arrive somewhat by choice when they say, one way or another, "No more." Emotions, not only in the dying but in those who love them, often include ambivalence, anticipatory loss, and tenderness—and darker ones, like caregiver burnout, horror at the ravages of illness, fear, reluctance to let go, and impatience for it all to be over.

No matter how uncertain the hour of death may still be, take a breath. Death is on its way. This is the time to prepare for the difficult labor of dying, just as the final trimester of pregnancy signals the time to get everything in place for the hard work of giving birth.

This will not be an individual journey. Although we ultimately die alone, we will need the help of others until our last moments. A good death is easier for people with family members or a strong network of friends to provide practical support, and a hospice or palliative care team to educate caregivers and handle pain and other symptoms. When basic needs for comfort, connection, and pain control are met, dying people often have the breathing space to address what concerns them, emotionally and spiritually. That requires accepting the coming of death, and making practical plans.

FINDING ALLIES IN HOSPICE

If you want to die at home, I suggest you arrange an informational meeting with a hospice, even if you think you're not sick enough yet. You should explore enrolling as soon as visiting a doctor becomes difficult, and any time you have uncontrolled pain. Hospice will usually be the most financially viable way to get the medical and practical care you need at home, with the best pain control, and the best preparations for a calm and peaceful death.

Hospices are widely misunderstood. It's tragic that half of those who enroll do so only two weeks before death, when they could have benefited for far longer. Many families say afterward that they wished they'd contacted hospice earlier. To clear up common confusions, I've compiled a list of myths about hospice and the realities you will find instead.

A hospice is a building.

Reality: The first modern hospice—St. Christopher's in London, founded in 1967—is indeed a residence for dying people. But in the United States, a "hospice" isn't usually a brick-and-mortar building, but a package of coordinated services reimbursed by health insurance. Hospice teams provide emotional, practical, medical, and spiritual support to terminally ill people and their families and friends. Their doctors, nurses, chaplains, social workers, physical therapists, and other professionals make house calls to wherever their patients are, including private homes, nursing homes, and hospitals. Some hospices are branches of national for-profit chains; others are novice mom-and-pop businesses; still others are local community nonprofits with years of experience, and these are often, but not always, the best. There are some residential hospices in the United States, but they're mostly funded by philanthropy, and therefore few and far between.

Hospice is bedside care for the last hours of life. To qualify, people must be a few days from death.

Reality: Medicare's hospice benefit is available to anyone within six months of dying, and some private insurance covers up to a year. People who get hospice care early in their disease often continue to work, see friends, and do what matters to them. Paradoxically, their well-being often immediately improves once they get good pain management, and less stressful, better-coordinated, medical care at home.

Signing up for hospice is signing your death warrant.

Reality: It's true that hospice patients must let go of their old doctors and give up cure-oriented treatments. But if a new treatment surfaces that you want to try, you can disenroll from hospice without penalty, get treated, and return when you want to. About 15 percent of people on hospice get healthy enough to disenroll, at least for a while. Saying the word "hospice" will not make anybody die faster.

Hospice is expensive.

Reality: Hospices provide, at no charge, hospital beds and supplies; nursing care in the home; medications for pain, breathlessness, and anxiety; doctors' visits and twenty-four-hour phone consultations. Their social workers and chaplains support caregivers, help resolve family conflicts, and can help you create a plan for a peaceful death. There are no co-pays. However, there are gaps. You'll have to pay out of pocket or do without treatments the hospice considers life-extending rather than palliative. If you're in a nursing home (technically known as a "skilled nursing facility," or SNF), you'll have to choose: Medicare will not pay simultaneously for both hospice services and skilled nursing, because SNF stays are supposed to be for rehabilitation. People in this bind usually keep the SNF benefit, which covers more care, and pay for hospice or physician house call services out of pocket, or ask doctors to provide palliative care or comfort care. Then they transfer to hospice for the final days of active dying.

Hospice covers round-the-clock home care.

Reality: Not so—and this is a major shortcoming. Insurance reimbursements for hospices have declined, all provide fewer services than they used to, and more are run as businesses rather than as altruistic community organizations. Team members make house calls lasting up to an hour or so, but they rarely spend hours in the home. Hands-on bedside care, including bathing, diaper-changing, giving medication, and feeding, must be provided by friends, family, or aides paid out of pocket. Medicaid will provide home health aides to those with limited incomes and savings of $2,000 or less; a hospice "benefits coordinator" can help you with the application. Sometimes nonprofit hospices with strong community ties can steer you to charitable grants that cover some home care or a residential hospice.

When someone is actively dying and family members become afraid, they are often shocked to call the hospice and discover that no staff member will rush to the bedside. Teams are often stretched thin, the precise hour of death is always unpredictable, and most hospices do not consider it part of their mission to be present at the moment of death. At the very least, hospices should be honest about what they will and won't do, and provide adequate reassurance to family members, along with a clear picture of what dying will be like. Look for a hospice with a staffing ratio of one nurse for every nine to fifteen patients: the lower the caseload, the greater the chance someone will come at short notice.

Hospices push morphine, addicting the dying and hastening their deaths.

Reality: Many previously held medical assumptions turn upside down when someone is dying, and this includes most of what you think you know about pain control and addiction. Thanks to the current addiction epidemic, we have learned to regard drugs like benzodiazepines, Valium, morphine, fentanyl, OxyContin, and methadone with deep suspicion. But for people on hospice, they can be godsends. Unaddressed pain and agitation are distressing to everyone, and can absorb all the attention of the person dying. (This is still the most common barrier to a peaceful death.) Hospice nurses are your best defense: they are more experienced than most doctors in skillful pain management.

The cautions surrounding opiates—that they're addictive and sometimes life-threatening—are very relevant for young people who are not dying, but have little meaning for the terminally ill. Addiction is not an issue for the dying. Pain is. Morphine is usually self-administered, and the amount taken (via tablets, a patch, an infusion pump, or a squirt under the tongue) is controlled by the dying person or those caring for them. Those on morphine for months can tolerate extremely high doses. When you are dying, there is no shame in being dependent on a drug that will control your pain and give you the mental freedom to say an adequate goodbye.

Because so many people don't enroll in hospice until a few days before death, family members sometimes mistakenly conclude that death was caused by a drug like morphine or fentanyl, rather than by the natural course of a fatal disease. Many people die *under the influence* of morphine, but very few die much faster *because of* it.

Only people with cancer qualify for hospice.

Reality: It is still harder than it should be to qualify, but it may be easier than you think. Two doctors, usually a personal physician and the hospice director, must sign a certificate saying they expect you to die within six months if your disease follows its normal course.

Twelve conditions automatically qualify, including stage four cancers, advanced heart failure, HIV-AIDS, kidney failure, liver failure, lung failure (COPD), ALS, and other rapidly fatal neurological diseases. Unfortunately, the list doesn't include dementia or the slow fade that nurses call "the dwindles," which aren't covered until their final stages. Formerly, people in their final declines were admitted under a vague, catch-all diagnosis called "failure to thrive." But Medicare removed it from the list after a 2013 *Washington Post* article exposed for-profit hospice chains that used it to aggressively enroll people who lived more than six months.

If a hospice rejects you, forget it.

Reality: If you're turned down by one hospice, ask why, and apply again as soon as health conditions worsen. Admission standards vary, and you may find one hospice more flexible than another. Molly Bourne, MD, the former medical director of Hospice by the Bay in Larkspur, California, enrolled about half of her patients on "a judgment call," after she documented accelerating decline. "They didn't meet the strict criteria, but I could tell you they were going to die soon," she said.

"Let's say someone has Alzheimer's but they're still walking and talking and therefore don't meet Medicare's standard criteria," said Dr. Bourne. "But they've been hospitalized three times in the past year with pneumonia, have lost five pounds in the last two months, and have gone from feeding themselves to not knowing how to use a spoon in the past three months. I can make the argument that this person is not going to be able to eat very soon, and they're going to be dead within six months. And I can tell you, I'm usually right."

Families should keep a detailed diary. "Really get the story straight before meeting with the [hospice] physician," said Dr. Bourne. "Families want to look optimistic, but they should remember how the patient was six months ago. Caregivers don't give themselves credit for all the stuff they're doing. You're saying she dresses herself, but you're the one picking out the clothes and making sure she doesn't fall, and you're not calculating that as needing assistance."

You are most likely to be admitted when you or your caregivers can document rapid loss of weight, muscle mass, and interest in food; growing fatigue and hours spent napping; repeated hospitalizations without improvement; and escalating difficulties with feeding, getting out of a chair, speaking, swallowing, walking, sitting up, smiling, or recognizing a relative.

NEXT STEPS

If you are nervous about hospice, I suggest beginning with an "informational meeting" or an "evaluation intake appointment." Think of yourself as conducting research, and separate that from your decision-making. If you like going online, you can compare local hospice ratings at the "Hospice Compare" page of Medicare's website. Ask around about friends' experiences, phone at least three hospices, and observe how you feel during the phone calls. Did you get the information you needed? Were you rushed or listened to? It won't make you die any faster to explore what hospice has to offer. You may even, like Mary Jane Denzer, feel better and live longer.

Are you still hoping to benefit from curative medicine, or reluctant to say goodbye to doctors who have helped you through difficult times? That's fine. Hospice won't cover their services, but you can pay out of pocket, or forgo hospice and get support from a physician house call program, or an outpatient palliative care or advanced illness management program—if you can find one.

If you forgo hospice, and a hospital continues to be your medical option of last resort, accept the fact that this may very well be the place where you die. You will face a different set of challenges to a peaceful and meaningful death; the next chapter will discuss how to bring a sense of the sacred into circumstances there.

But beware: dying in a hospital can be traumatic to the dying and to their survivors. Avoid it if you can. Survivors of people who die in an ICU suffer higher rates of depression, post-traumatic stress, and prolonged, complicated grieving. In the words of Anna Reisman, director of the Humanities in Medicine program at Yale School of Medicine, "[It is a] bizarre fact that most hospital deaths are handled by the youngest and least-experienced doctors." Saving lives is a hospital's specialty. Supporting a good death rarely is.

SETTLING YOUR AFFAIRS

What matters most to people given the strange gift of knowing that death is on its way? Emergency medical technician Matthew O'Reilly of Long Island has attended many people dying by the side of the highway after fatal car accidents, trapped in mangled automobiles. In a memorable TED talk, he said that he'd decided early on in his career it was "not my place to comfort the dying with my lies." When gravely injured people ask him for the truth, he tells them they're dying. Their eyes, he says, almost universally reflect calm and acceptance. But most have three pieces of unfinished business. They have regrets and want to be forgiven. They fear they'll be forgotten and hope they'll be remembered. And they want to know that their lives had meaning.

Ask yourself: What stands in the way, right now, of your dying in peace? What do you regret? What do you fear? What does a "good death" mean to you? Do you want to know how people with your particular illness tend to die, and what can be done to ease your symptoms? Are there certain friends and relatives whom you *don't* want to see? What might help your survivors feel at ease after you're gone?

Your to-do list may be as practical as deciding which family member will get a favorite vase, and putting the name on the bottom of it. It may be as creative as writing or talking about what you contributed during your precious human life. And it may be as intimate as talking about your fears, expressing gratitude and love, asking for and granting forgiveness, and saying goodbye.

Here are some examples of what others have done when they sensed, or were told, that they were approaching the end of life. Broadly speaking, these tasks can be sorted into three categories: arranging practicalities; telling your story; and completing the interpersonal work of life's end.

Practicalities. After he was diagnosed with advanced cancer, rancher Jim Modini and his wife, Shirley, bequeathed their ranch to an environmental group and made sure that loving, competent caregivers were in place to care for Shirley, who had dementia, after Jim was gone.

Telling Your Story. Jane Sidwell's father, Clarence Welgos, was diagnosed with esophageal cancer when he was seventy-two. He'd been a radioman on battleships in the Pacific Ocean during the Second World War. In the extensive diary he kept during those years, he referred frequently to the "horrors" he'd lived through, but he never talked about them to his family. After his diagnosis, he took out his war uniform and reviewed his World War II scrapbook, diary, and photos. He also sought out another veteran and together they held long conversations about their war experiences. He spent months creating an annotated map of the Pacific Ocean, charting the courses of the battleships he'd served on and naming all his commanders and the major battles he'd lived through. The map still hangs in his widow's den. It is one of the ways that he will be remembered.

Saying Goodbye. A year before he died of cirrhosis of the liver at the age of seventy-two (caused by medications to treat the effects of a war injury), Jack Dempsey, a retired teacher who'd recently been widowed, moved from Kentucky to a small town in North Dakota to be near his daughter Jackie. As he and Jackie, who was in her forties, drove northward with his things, he asked her to detour through southern Illinois, where he'd been raised. They stopped in little towns where he'd grown up and paid visits to long-lost cousins, uncles, and aunts. "It was heartbreakingly sad yet joyful to see how he was welcomed with open arms by all of these, to me, seemingly ancient relatives," Jackie remembers. Jack visited his father's grave, and tried, without success, to find the graves of his mother and his baby sister in a vast, unattended cemetery. "He was saying hello but he was also saying goodbye. I didn't see that then," Jackie said, "but I see it in retrospect."

Six months later, her father weakened dramatically and was admitted to hospice. Jackie and her husband moved her father into their house in Minot, North Dakota, where his hospital bed had a view of the river Souris. For months, as he grew steadily weaker and more confused, Jack spent his days looking out and marveling at the river and the colors of the trees and the sky. One day, as Jackie was sitting by his bedside holding his hand, he looked toward the river and said, "It's so far over that lake. I'm not sure I can make it."

"Where are you going, Dad?" she asked him.

"I have to go home. I have to get over that lake but I don't think I can make it."

"I'll help you," she said. "I will help you get to the other side of the lake." He died of pneumonia a week later.

CHOOSING THE TIME OF DEATH

More than 58 million Americans—those living on the West Coast, or in Hawaii, Montana, Oregon, Vermont, or the District of Columbia—may now legally obtain death-hastening prescriptions when they are terminally ill. Until recently, this practice was criminalized in most developed countries, and the Hippocratic Oath forbids it. But it isn't new: throughout history, some medical professionals have quietly hastened death when they believed that their moral obligation to relieve suffering overrode a blanket duty to prolong life.

Among them is one of the most admired people in western medical history: the microbiologist Louis Pasteur, the father of the germ theory of disease, the inventor of pasteurization, and the developer of inoculations for rabies. In the mid-1880s, at the Hotel Dieu, a famous Parisian hospital, Pasteur treated five Russian farmers, all of whom had been bitten by the same rabid wolf and were dying horrible, protracted deaths. When they did not respond to Pasteur's new serum, the farmers pleaded to be put out of their misery.

Pasteur conferred with the hospital's head pharmacist, who compounded a lethal prescription, which the farmers took of their own volition. They died almost immediately. Pasteur's actions may have been merciful, but they were devastating to all who observed them: a silence fell over the ward, wrote the novelist Léon Daudet, who was there studying medicine. He and his fellow doctors, he wrote, "cried tears of horror. We were at the end of our nerves, annihilated."

More than a century later, 12 million people watched a You-Tube video made in 2014 by Brittany Maynard, a beautiful young California teacher who wanted to cut short the final ravages of her brain cancer but could not do so legally in her home state. She moved to Oregon, which has allowed physician-assisted dying since 1997, and took legally prescribed lethal drugs there.

Planned, voluntarily timed deaths like hers can be as calm, poignant, and sacred as any other. Brittany's husband and step-father were with her as she died, while her mother read aloud her daughter's favorite poem, "The Summer Day" by Mary Oliver. It includes the famous lines,

> Doesn't everything die at last, and too soon?
> Tell me, what is it you plan to do
> with your one wild and precious life?

Maynard's video created a groundswell of support for expanding the right to time one's death, which was legalized two years later in California. This pathway to the end of life is heavily regulated wherever it is legal, and it is available only to people certified to be of sound mind and within six months of dying. Health systems may opt out of cooperating, and many, especially Catholic ones, do. It is of no use to the demented, or to people with physical limitations that prevent them from taking a drug without practical help. (Those with such conditions must decide early in the disease process, and sometimes cannot qualify at all.) Others hasten death informally by fasting, known as voluntary stopping of eating and drinking, or VSED. The practice was familiar in classical Greece, where the stoic Greek philosopher Cleanthes stopped eating for a few days at his doctor's suggestion to heal an ulcer, decided not to start up again, and brought on his own death at the age of ninety-nine. Dying occurs relatively painlessly by dehydration, as long as nothing *at all* is consumed, and typically takes ten to fourteen days. This ancient practice is currently allowed in every state: there is no law requiring people to eat or to be force-fed.

Alan Alberts of Bellingham, Washington, a computer consul-tant, was seventy-five when he was diagnosed with the early stages of Alzheimer's disease in 2011. He'd watched his mother die an agonizingly slow death on a locked "memory" unit. In 2013, while he could still make his own medical decisions, he chose to stop eating and drinking, with the support of his wife, Phyllis Shacter. As Phyllis described in her 2017 book *Choosing to Die*, the couple arranged for supportive caregivers and consulted a lawyer and a sympathetic doctor. Phyllis created an altar at home where candles burned continuously for the eight days it took Alan to die.

In midweek, a social worker from the county's elder abuse department came to the house, most likely alerted by a former paid caregiver who was uncomfortable with what the couple was doing. Phyllis pulled out her well-organized legal documents to demonstrate that Alan was following his own wishes and had the right to do so. The social worker was satisfied, and Alan continued to a quiet death.

Others hasten death outside the law, sometimes with the help of a volunteer group called the Final Exit Network. Sometimes family and friends are informed and cooperative, and the dying hold a farewell party or otherwise say goodbye. A dear man whom I knew through a meditation group, and whom I shall call Phillip, was eighty-nine when he ended his life this way, with the knowledge of his wife, brother, and closest friends. A former air force pilot, athlete, and inspired teacher, he was miserable, losing weight rapidly, bent over a walker, and increasingly isolated by deafness and cognitive impairment that had worsened dramatically after a heart valve replacement surgery. After spending his last week saying goodbye to those closest to him, he ate applesauce to combat nausea and took a hundred hoarded, legally prescribed Seconal pills, following directions in the book *Final Exit*. His brother, who was with him, left immediately afterward, and Phillip's wife, Aida, returned to her unconscious husband's bedside for the five hours it took him to die, singing him songs they'd loved, like "Old Devil Moon" and "My One and Only Love."

The couple had not consulted a lawyer or doctor or planned

for the aftermath, and after Phillip died, Aida called 911 to have her husband pronounced dead. The local coroner and sheriff's deputies converged on the house and questioned her for three and a half hours. She pretended she'd known nothing of her husband's plans, and was silent about the involvement of his brother. (Promoting or assisting a suicide is a crime in California, as it is in most states.) "They wanted to know what he'd eaten that morning, and what he'd talked about," she said. "Why had I not known? Why was he sleeping in the guest room?" Aida continued to profess ignorance. "I didn't know I could lie like this!" she said. "It was an awful feeling, but I had to make sense and protect his brother."

Some people in poor health try to end their lives on their own, without involving family. They have often fallen through cracks in the health system: sick enough to be miserable, not sick enough for hospice, and without practical support or home-based palliative care. Dying this way is not illegal, but having been privy to two botched attempts, I don't recommend it. The people I knew were discovered and resuscitated. Their advance directives were disregarded, they were placed in intensive care units, and they lost the right to make their own medical decisions until they were deemed to no longer be depressed or a threat to themselves. If you are considering this path, please speak to someone about your despair and your plans. Taking one's life without the knowledge and acceptance of family or friends often leaves trauma in its wake. A palliative care or hospice team may find ways to make things better. The National Suicide Prevention hotline number is 1-800-273-8255. Please call it.

LOVING, THANKING, AND FORGIVING

Hospice nurses like Redwing Keyssar often say that people die as they've lived. Whether you are a caregiver or a dying person, please don't use the suggestions in this book as standards to force yourself or others to meet. Some people get ready for death watching a Red Sox game and eating pizza.

Nevertheless, many people intuitively complete some version of five emotional tasks of the end of life, popularized by the pioneering hospice doctor Ira Byock in these simple words: "Please forgive me. I forgive you. Thank you. I love you. Goodbye." This important work doesn't have to be done out loud. Nor does it even require openly acknowledging that you are, or someone you love is, approaching the end of life.

After my father had his first major stroke, I began writing him what I later called "legacy letters." I thanked him for reading me *The Story of Babar: The Little Elephant* when I was tiny, and for teaching me to read and to swim. We spent a year exchanging letters and photographs this way, recalling the many happy hours we'd spent during my early childhood. I didn't have to say aloud that I knew he was approaching the end of his life, or that we were indirectly healing the rifts of my aggrieved adolescence and beyond, but we tacitly understood. He closed one of his last letters to me with, "You must think of this often, because it will sustain you." It still does.

Do not underestimate the power of your emotional legacy, expressed in even a small, last-minute exchange within a difficult relationship. Kathy Duby was raised on the East Coast by a violent alcoholic mother. Kathy had no memory of ever hearing her mother say "I love you." Kathy eventually moved to California, and decades went by. The two women's relationship continued to be marked by bitterness, distrust, and estrangement.

When Kathy was in her forties, her mother, then in her seventies, developed breast cancer. The disease metastasized despite surgery, chemotherapy, and radiation. A little more than a week before her death, her mother was admitted to the hospital. Over the phone, she said to her daughter Kathy, "Don't come. I don't want to see you." Kathy got on a plane on the advice of a friend who told her that if she didn't fly back, she would regret it for the rest of her life.

Kathy walked into her mother's hospital room. There she found a tiny figure curled up in a hospital bed—"shrunken, yellow, bald, bronzed by jaundice," as she later described it in a poem. This was the mother she had feared for so long. The two women looked at each other in silence. Kathy's mother said aloud, for the first time that Kathy could remember, "I love you. I'm sorry." That was it.

Kathy replied, "I love you and I'm sorry."

"Those few moments," said Kathy, "cleared up a lifetime of misunderstanding each other."

When you think of how you'd like your own death to go, I suggest you make plans for the basics—comfort, adequate help, and pain control—and then expand your horizons. One man dying of multiple sclerosis in a nursing home, who'd formerly worked as a forester, was gurneyed out into the woods by volunteer firefighters for a last view of his beloved trees. In Australia, paramedics have taken dying people to the beach for a few minutes to gaze at the ocean or to lick an ice cream cone, before delivering them to the hospital. One of my closest friends will never forget the look on her dying mother's face when she cued up Frank Sinatra on her mother's headphones.

Are there particular words you'd like to hear that might help you die in peace? Might you need reassurance, for instance, that a vulnerable family member will be taken care of? One agitated man, who'd made his living putting up holiday decorations on the Main Streets of several towns, died peacefully after his hospice nurse told him that the season was over and all the decorations were put away.

GETTING HELP FROM YOUR TRIBE

Coming together to help someone prepare for and experience a good death, just as our ancestors did, is a rite of passage worth reviving. Everyone benefits, as long as caregiving burdens are spread widely enough, because helping others makes people feel better about themselves. For those without substantial assets or Medicaid, most bedside care will be provided by friends, volunteers, and relatives, as has been done for centuries. The excellent handbook *Share the Care* shows ways to divvy up tasks so that people do what they're good at, get satisfaction from it, and don't burn out.

Share the Care suggests picking an organizer to convene a face-to-face meeting of everyone interested in helping out. At that meeting, those involved can parcel out tasks, including a hands-on point person who can live in the home or nearby; someone to coordinate volunteers, using an online calendar or a website like LotsaHelpingHands.org; and someone to match volunteers with the types of help they're best at (shopping, running errands, bedside caregiving, or researching outside sources of help like public benefits and community groups). The most critical role to fill is that of a health care agent, if one hasn't been chosen yet—someone to make sure that appropriate and wanted medical care is delivered (including pain management); that end-of-life paperwork is up to date; and that when the time comes, all unwanted or painful medical treatments are stopped.

Don't turn down even the smallest offer of help. When my former dance teacher, Stephanie Moore, was diagnosed with ovarian cancer, her daughter and dozens of people she knew took care of her round the clock for five months. Tall and blond, and possessed of extraordinary energy, drive, and talent, Stephanie was divorced and lived alone and on a shoestring. But she was rich in social connections. When she was weakened by cancer, surgery, and chemotherapy, and unable to drive or shop, she drew on the deep "gratitude bank" she'd built over decades of teaching writing and dance classes, and in her membership in a recovery program. Whenever anybody said, "Let me know if you need anything!" Stephanie would whip out her calendar; she always had an answer.

Her daughter was there every day. Another well-organized woman with a full-time job handled the calendar of helpers online in the evenings. I used to bring a chicken dinner to share on Monday nights, while others took regular four-hour weekly shifts to keep her company. Because the commitments were shared and well organized, no single person was overwhelmed. Those who showed up were not necessarily those she expected; some close friends didn't come much, while others who barely knew her drew deep satisfaction from being part of her support team.

My husband, Brian, drove Stephanie to her chemotherapy sessions and slept in a sleeping bag on the floor by her bed on the many nights when she was afraid to be alone. When she had trouble breathing in her last two months, he also paid for oxygen equipment that her health plan refused to provide.

Stephanie insisted until her last week that she was going to beat her cancer. She tried, unsuccessfully, to get the "maximum chemo," which her doctors said would kill her. She was particular about how she wanted things done, and she refused the support of hospice until a couple of weeks before her death. She spent her last three days in a hospital because she became too agitated and delusional to be adequately cared for in her own home.

She was in her mid-fifties when she died, with many ambitions and yearnings unfulfilled—to publish a novel she'd written, and to once again be in a committed, loving relationship. Nothing about her dying was easy. Those who cared for her could not make her peaceful. But shortly before she entered the hospital, she invited Brian and some of her closest friends to help her plan her funeral. And after she died, everyone who helped her could look back with pride on the job they did.

Ways to Prepare:

- Call a hospice for an informational meeting, even if you don't think you're sick enough yet. Ask yourself what stands in the way of your dying in peace, and work to address it.
- Consider the five emotional tasks of dying: thank you, I love you, please forgive me, I forgive you, and goodbye.
- Enlarge your circle of support. Convene a meeting and assign roles.

CHAPTER 7

Active Dying

The Tree Needs to Come Down • This Is What Dying Looks Like
Preparing for a Home Death • Preparing in a Nursing Home
Giving Care • The Final Hours • Humanizing a Hospital Death
Improvising Rites of Passage • Welcoming Mystery
Saying Goodbye

Late Fragment

And did you get what
You wanted from this life, even so?
I did.
And what did you want?
To call myself beloved, to feel myself
Beloved on the earth.

—RAYMOND CARVER, written not long before his death in 1988

You are, or someone you love is, likely to find this chapter helpful if you are within a few weeks or days of dying, as shown by several of the following signs.

The gravely ill person:

- Stops eating.
- Talks about needing to pack, "go home," cross a river, or move to a higher floor of a nursing home.
- "Sees," dreams of, or speaks of attending a party with the dead.
- Talks of wanting to join dead loved ones.
- Sees spirit guides, such as a coyote, the Virgin Mary, or something more idiosyncratic, like a man in a top hat sitting on the roof outside the window.
- Cannot get out of bed. Needs to be helped to the bathroom, or uses a diaper.
- Says "I'm dying" or "There isn't much time."
- "Rallies," reviving briefly with a burst of joy, exuberance, and expressions of love that may last several hours or occasionally days, followed by a collapse of energy.
- Withdraws, naps for hours, speaks little, and keeps eyes closed.

If you, or someone you love, is dying in a hospital, these common-sense harbingers may be obscured by a hubbub of medical technologies. In that case, look for the following signs:

- Being in an ICU with stage four cancer or with sepsis, a catastrophic whole-body response to infection. The older and more fragile the person, and the greater the number of coexisting serious illnesses, prior hospital stays, and prior days in the ICU, the more likely it is that death is close.
- Having ICU doctors argue about treatment, order dialysis, or speak of "multiple organ systems failure," often code language for "dying" or a predictor of its imminent arrival.
- Having a doctor suggest meeting with a palliative care or hospice team, or talk about "goals of care," "discontinuing life support," or "withdrawing care." These sometimes insensitive phrases mean they think it's time to shift from fighting death to relieving suffering, providing comfort care, and preparing for the best possible death.

THE TREE NEEDS TO COME DOWN

Modern death takes many shapes. Arranging a peaceful one poses different challenges in a private home, a nursing home, and a hospital. Nevertheless, most deaths share a few simple commonalities, notably the need for physical comfort, human connection, and pain control. All are easier to provide when death is anticipated. But dying has become so hidden, medically drawn out, and ambiguous that many of us no longer trust our gut sense that it is on its way. Experienced doctors, aides, and hospice nurses tend to be more attuned, but they have learned never to precisely predict the moment of death, and they, too, sometimes miss its harbingers. Only in retrospect did Diana, a former social worker who serves as a paid companion for aging people, recognize the signs shown by one of her favorite clients, a retired engineer named Gordon Lechenger.

Gordon was ninety-six and lived in an apartment in a luxurious assisted living complex in a small town in Minnesota. In the six years that Diana served as his companion and aide, their relationship evolved from an employer-employee transaction to an intimate, reciprocal friendship. Gordon was a widower with two loving daughters and several granddaughters and great-grandchildren, the kind of man who during the winter holidays would ask the staff at his residence what they were buying for their children. He regularly dressed in suits, ties and hats, and Diana remembers him as "very nice-looking, a dapper man, a gentleman. The kind of man who would open doors for you and feel good about it."

Diana first met him when he was in his mid-eighties, after he injured his shoulder. She was hired by his daughters to help him dress, and to drive him in his big leased car to tour the countryside, to visit art fairs, and to go to an old-line department store, where he'd buy new shirts and hats and schmooze with the staff. Sometimes he'd ask her to Google something—like who invented the fork?—and then talk about it with his fellow residents at dinner.

Gordon could read Diana's face. If she came to work looking stressed about her own family, he'd say, "Lock the door. I'm turning my collar around," meaning he was about to play priest. He would hold her hand and look into her eyes, and when she finished unburdening herself, he'd say gently, "This, too, shall pass."

Over the next decade, a heart attack and repeated hospitalizations and injuries left him weak and fragile. He gradually stopped walking and relied more and more on a wheelchair.

The first sign of his approaching death followed a brief hospitalization for unexplained stomach bleeding. After he stabilized, he went to a skilled nursing home, paid for by Medicare, where he had to share a room. When he learned from his daughters that he had run out of money and could no longer afford to return to his expensive assisted living apartment, Diana saw him change markedly. Previously, he'd thrown himself into physical therapy. This time, he refused to go.

One morning at the nursing home, Diana found him looking out the window at a majestic old oak tree. He told her that the tree "needed to come down" because it was old and had "had a good life." Sometimes he'd get a faraway look in his eyes and when Diana asked, he'd tell her that he was remembering dancing with his dead wife, Angela. When Diana got ready to leave for a month to care for her sick mother-in-law in Australia, Gordon barely responded—a lack of interest in her affairs that was totally out of character. His withdrawal, his reminiscing about the dead, and his speaking in metaphors about the natural cycle of life and death, were all foreshadowings.

When Diana returned, Gordon was no longer listless and preoccupied with the past. "He looked at me with such brightness and joy," Diana said. "Never in my life had anybody looked at me that way."

It was a warm spring day. She took him for a walk in his wheelchair and then to a St. Patrick's Day party in the activities room. Everything he encountered filled him with joy. Normally reserved and dignified, he happily wore a green cardboard hat decorated with a shamrock, tapped his feet to Irish music, called the crab cakes "delicious," and laughed at the Irish jokes Diana downloaded from the Internet. This burst of joy, this final spilling-over of life energy, this gratitude for the world, this letting go of restraint, was the harbinger that hospice nurses call "rallying."

The next morning, Diana found Gordon in bed, trembling. His doctor made a house call, decided that Gordon had a cold, and reassured his daughters that it was safe for the extended family to take their planned Florida vacation.

The next day Diana found Gordon sitting in his armchair, looking ashen. He said with uncharacteristic abruptness, "You are just in time."

His lower back, he told her, was hurting badly. She called an aide, and together they moved him back to bed. The aide gave him Tylenol. It did nothing for him.

The next four hours were among the most difficult of Diana's life.

Uncontrolled pain is a common barrier to a peaceful death, currently affecting 61 percent of people in their last year of life. It is most frequently endured when death comes unexpectedly, without the expert pain management usually provided by a hospice. Gordon, who was usually stoic, kept shifting in bed, trying to get comfortable. Diana rearranged his pillows and called nursing staff, but getting medical authorization for a stronger painkiller was agonizingly slow. An hour passed. She sat on the bed and tried to reach under Gordon's back to rub it. "The dear man attempted to move over to make it easier for me, which he was too weak to do," she said. "He was such a kind soul."

In the meantime, Gordon's roommate, lying behind a curtain in the next bed, and sensing perhaps that death was near, turned on his television, and then turned it up louder. Another hour passed.

A young nurse came in with a big pain pill and handed it to Gordon with a glass of water. After he swallowed it, the young woman set down the glass and quickly walked out. As the television blared behind the curtain, Gordon's breathing grew ragged. A more experienced nurse came in, asked if Gordon had a do-not-resuscitate order, learned that he did, and said to Diana, "He doesn't look good. Just hold his hands." Diana held him. Gordon choked, took two final breaths, and stopped breathing. Diana believes he had waited to die until she returned.

Because so few of us are exposed to dying as a normal life passage, we are both captivated and tyrannized by death. We are either terrified into silence and avoidance, or we flee into a sentimental narrative of the "good death," a purely spiritual experience where all is forgiven, the heavens open, and the secretions, smells, exhaustion, and messiness disappear. But a death, like a birth, weds the animal to the soulful. Perhaps a more realistic hope for caregivers, and for ourselves when we are dying, is for a "good-enough death," where we keep the dying as comfortable and pain free as possible, and leave room for the beautiful and the transcendent, which may or may not occur.

The final letting-go is an inexorable physical process, akin to giving birth. Vital organs shut down one after another or all at once, starved of oxygen, nutrients, and energy. Breathing becomes ragged, lips and toes turn blue, awareness turns inward, the dying person stops responding to others, and sinks into a deep, sleep-like coma before taking a few final breaths. This stage, which hospice nurses call "active dying," usually lasts three to eight days, but sometimes less and sometimes more.

Sometimes dying is gentle all the way to the end, and sometimes not. Moments of fear, agitation, confusion, breathlessness, irritability, anger and pain are normal, and although they can often be soothed medically, dying can be wrenching for the dying, and exhausting and distressing to those who are with them.

Keep your heart open and your expectations low. "I don't tell families at the outset that their experience can be life-affirming, and leave them with positive feelings and memories," said hospice nurse Jerry Soucy. "I say instead that we're going to do all we can to make the best of a difficult situation, because that's what we confront. The positive feelings sometimes happen in the moment, but are more likely to be of comfort in the days and months after a death."

Even if you find yourself looking after a dying person without hospice or experienced help, you and those who love you can do this. The presence of a single calm person in the room can make a tremendous difference. People have been dying, and sitting by the bedsides of the dying, for millennia. If you are a caregiver, the most important thing to do is to take your cues from the dying person, and imagine what you'd want if you were in that bed. Having a map of what you are likely to encounter may help you to manage your own fears and to understand that what you are seeing, while difficult, is normal.

Dying is not an emergency. You can prepare for it, you can cooperate with it, and you can draw on wells of fortitude and love that you may not know existed within you. Dying people and those who sit with them have borne many difficult things. They've climbed mountains, built businesses, nurtured children, and lived through chronic illness, loneliness, marriage, divorce, and bereavement. Now comes the final labor of leaving this earth. At times it will be an ordeal. Much will be out of your control. But expressing your caring is never fruitless, and you may look back with pride on how you helped.

THIS IS WHAT DYING LOOKS LIKE

You don't have to be a saint to die well at home. You do have to have people who love you. John Masterson was an artist and sign painter, the ninth of ten children born to a devout Catholic couple in Davenport, Iowa. His mother died when he was eight, and he and two of his sisters spent nearly a year in an orphanage. He moved to Seattle in his twenties, earned a black belt in karate, started a sign-painting business, and converted to Soka Gakkai, a branch of Buddhism whose primary practice is chanting. He never left his house without intoning three times in Japanese, *Nam-myoho-renge-kyo* (I honor the impeccable teachings of the Lotus Sutra).

John was fifty-seven and living alone, without health insurance, when he developed multiple myeloma, an incurable blood cancer. He didn't have much money: he was the kind of person who would spend hours teaching a fellow artist how to apply gold leaf, while falling behind on his paid work. But thanks to his large extended family, his karate practice, and his fierce dedication to his religion, he was part of several tribes. He was devoted to his three children— each the result of a serious relationship with a different woman— and they loved him equally fiercely. His youngest sister, Anne, a nurse who had followed him to Seattle, said he had "an uncanny ability to piss people off but make them love him loyally forever."

When he first started feeling exhausted and looking gaunt, John tried to cure himself with herbs and chanting. By the time Anne got him to a doctor, he had a tumor the size of a half grapefruit protruding from his breastbone. Myeloma is sometimes called a "smoldering" cancer because it can lie dormant for years. By the time John's was diagnosed, his was in flames.

Huge plasma cells were piling up in his bone marrow, while other rogue blood cells dissolved bone and dumped calcium into his bloodstream, damaging his kidneys and brain function. He grew too weak and confused to work or drive. Bills piled up and his house fell into foreclosure. Anne, who worked the evening shift at a local hospital, moved him into her house and drove him to various government offices to apply for food stamps, Social Security disability, and Medicaid. She would frequently get up early to stand in line outside social services offices with his paperwork in a portable plastic file box.

Medicaid paid for the drug thalidomide, which cleared the calcium from John's bloodstream and helped his brain and kidneys recover. A blood-cancer specialist at the University of Washington Medical Center told him that a bone marrow transplant might buy him time, perhaps even years. But myeloma eventually returns; the transplant doesn't cure it. The treatment would temporarily destroy his immune system, could kill him, and would require weeks of recovery in sterile isolation. John decided against it, and was equally adamant that he'd never go on dialysis.

After six months on thalidomide, John recovered enough to move into a government-subsidized studio apartment near Pike Place Market. He loved being on his own again and wandered the market making videos of street musicians, which he'd post on Facebook. But Anne now had to drive across town to shop, cook, and clean for him.

The health plateau lasted more than a year. But by the fall of

2010, John could no longer bear one of thalidomide's most difficult side effects, agonizing neuropathic foot pain. When he stopped taking the drug, he knew that calcium would once again build up in his bloodstream, and that he was turning toward his death.

An older sister and brother flew out from Iowa to help Anne care for him. One sibling would spend the night, and another sibling, or John's oldest daughter Keely, a law student, would spend the day.

Christmas came and went. His sister Irene returned to Iowa and was replaced by another Iowa sister, Dottie, a devout Catholic. In early January, John developed a urinary tract infection and became severely constipated and unable to pee. Anne took him to the University of Washington medical center for what turned out to be the last time. His kidneys were failing and his bones were so eaten-away by disease that when he sneezed he broke several ribs. Before he left the hospital, John met with a hematologist, a blood specialist, who asked Anne to step briefly out of the room.

Anne does not know exactly what was said. But most UW doctors are well trained in difficult conversations, thanks to a morally responsible institutional culture on end-of-life issues. Doctors at UW do not simply present patients with retail options, like items on a menu, and expect them to blindly pick. Its doctors believe they have an obligation to use their clinical experience to act in their patients' best interests, and they are not afraid of making frank recommendations against futile and painful end-of-life treatments. When the meeting was over, the doctor told Anne that her brother "wanted to let nature take its course." He would enroll in hospice. Anne drove him home.

John knew he was dying. He told Anne that he wanted to "feel everything" about the process, even the pain. "He took this Buddhist perspective that if he suffered he would wipe out his bad karma. I said, 'Nah, that's just bullshit. You've done nothing wrong. The idea that we're sinners or have to suffer is ludicrous.'" She looked her brother in the eye. She knew she was going to be dispensing his medications when he no longer could, and she wasn't going to let him suffer. She told him, "You're not going to have a choice."

Anne said she "set an intention" not to resist her brother's dying, but to give him the most gentle death possible and to just let things unfold. On January 15, her birthday, she and John and a gaggle of other family members walked down to Pike Place Market to get a coffee and celebrate. John could barely walk. Anne kept close to him so that she could grab him if he fell. It was the last time he left the house.

The next morning, a Sunday, while Anne was sitting with John at his worktable, he looked out the window and asked her, "Do you think I'll die today?" Anne said, "Well, Sundays are good days to die, but no, I don't think it's today." It was the last fully coherent conversation she had with him.

He spent most of his last nine days in bed, as his kidneys failed and he grew increasingly confused. He didn't seem afraid, but he was sometimes grumpy. He had increasing difficulty finding words and craved celery, which he called "the green thing." He would ask Anne to take him to the bathroom, and then forget what he was supposed to do there. His daughter Keely took a leave of absence from law school, and Anne did the same from her job at the hospital. Fellow artists, fellow chanters, former students to whom he'd taught karate, nephews, nieces, and sign-painting clients visited, and Anne would prop him up on pillows to greet them.

Anne managed things, but with a light hand. She didn't vet visitors, and they came at all hours. If she needed to change his sheets or turn him, she would ask whoever was there to help her, and show them how. That way, she knew that other people were capable of caring for him when she wasn't there. "The ones that have the hardest time [with death] wring their hands and think they don't know what to do," she said. "But we *do* know what to do. Just think: *If it were my body, what would I want?* One of the worst things, when we're grieving, is the sense that *I didn't do enough*," she said. "But if you get in and help, you won't have that sense of helplessness."

Each day John ate and spoke less and slept more, until he lost consciousness and stopped speaking entirely. To keep him from developing bedsores, Anne would turn him from one side to the other every two hours, change his diaper if necessary, and clean him, with the help of whoever was in the room. He'd groan when she moved him, so about a half an hour beforehand, she'd crush morphine and Ativan pills, mix them with water as the hospice nurse had shown her, and drip them into John's mouth.

One morning Anne's distraught older brother accused her of "killing" John by giving him too much morphine—a common fear among relatives, who sometimes can't bear to up the dose as pain gets worse. At that moment, the hospice nurse arrived by chance, and calmly and gently explained, "Your brother is dying, and this is what dying looks like."

The death was communal. People flowed in and out, night and day, talking of what they loved about John and the things that annoyed them, bringing food, flowers, candles, and photographs until John's worktable looked like a crowded altar. Buddhists lit incense and chanted. Someone set up a phone tree, someone else made arrangements with a funeral home, and one of the Buddhists planned the memorial service.

Most of the organizing, however, fell to Anne. It may take a village to die well, but it also takes one strong person willing to take ownership—the human equivalent of the central pole holding up a circus tent. In the final two weeks, she was in almost superhuman motion. She leaned, she said, "into an element of the universe that knows more than I know. I was making it up as I went along. People contributed and it became very rich.

"That's not to say there weren't times when it was phenomenally stressful. I was dealing with all the logistics, and my own mixed emotions about my brother. I was flooded with memories of our very complicated relationship, and at the same time knowing that my intention was that he be laid to rest in the most gentle way possible."

Hospice was a quiet support in the background. Over the two years of his illness, John's care had perfectly integrated the medical and the practical, shifting seamlessly from prolonging his life and improving his functioning—as thalidomide and the doctors at UW had done—to relieving his suffering and attending his dying—as the hospice nurses and those who loved him had done. There were no demons under the bed or angels above the headboard. Nor were there beeping monitors and high-tech machines. His dying was labor intensive, as are most home deaths, and it was not without conflict.

A few days before he died, two of John's Iowa siblings beseeched Anne to call a priest to give John last rites in the Catholic Church. "It was a point of love for my siblings. They were concerned that John was going to burn in hell," Anne said. "But John hated priests." In tears, Anne called the Seattle church that handled such requests, and the priest, after a brief conversation, asked her to put Anne's sister on the phone. Yes, the sister acknowledged, John was a Buddhist. No, he hadn't requested the sacraments. Yes, his children were adamantly opposed. No, the priest told her, under the circumstances, he couldn't come. It wasn't John's wish.

Ten days after the family's last walk through Pike Place Market, the hospice nurse examined John early one morning and said, "He won't be here tomorrow." She was seeing incontrovertible physical signs: John's lips and fingertips were blue and mottled. He hadn't opened his eyes in days. His breathing was labored and irregular, but still oddly rhythmic, and he looked peaceful. The hospice nurse left. Anne, helped by John's daughter Keely and his sister Dottie, washed and turned John and gave him his meds. Then they sat by his side.

"It was January in Seattle," Anne said. "The sun was coming through the window and we could hear the market below beginning to wake up. We were just the three of us, talking and sharing our stories about him and the things we loved and didn't love, the things that had pissed us off but now we laughed about. I can't ever, in words, express the sweetness of that moment.

"He just had this one-room apartment with a little half-wall before the kitchen. I walked over to put water on to make coffee, and Keely said, 'his breathing's changed.'" Anne stopped, ran over, sat on the bed, and lifted her brother to a sitting position. He was light. She held him close, and during his last three breaths she chanted *Nam-myoho-renge-kyo,* as her brother had always done, three times, whenever he left his house. "I was really almost mouth-to-mouth chanting, and he died in my arms," she said. "We just held him, and then my sister Dottie said her prayers over him."

Anne sat next to her brother and said, "John, I did well."

"I know he would not have been able to orchestrate it any better than how it unfolded," she said. "It was a profound experience for me. I realized what a good death could be."

PREPARING FOR A HOME DEATH

When I first began this book, I expected to enthusiastically recommend hospice at home for everyone. I still think it's the best option for those who want to die at home and have the money for hired caregiving or a "tribe" to look after them. But after talking to many people who've attended difficult hospice deaths, I've realized that current gaps in hospice services put a good home death out of reach of many people. As I've said, hospice staff don't provide practical caregiving, and sometimes they're not available when family members panic, don't give enough morphine to control pain, or are otherwise overwhelmed.

Some people fall through the cracks because, even though they are dying and could benefit from comfort-focused medical care at home, they don't have the "right" diagnosis: a disease that moves quickly enough to qualify them for hospice as soon as they need it. Others live in neighborhoods where keeping narcotics at home will expose them to burglary, and where local pharmacies don't stock certain drugs for the same reason. Many single people don't have (or have outlived) the deep network of friends or relatives needed to make a long dying at home comfortable. For them, a better alternative may be a residential hospice, a nursing home or an assisted living residence friendly to hospice, or even a hospital.

If you have the resources for a home death, here are some suggestions—gathered from hospice nurses, family caregivers, and volunteers—for preparing yourself.

Plan ahead for the basic needs of the dying and those caring for them. That means food for vigilers and physical comfort for the dying person. (Once active dying begins, people will be too overwhelmed to go shopping.) Next, arrange medical care that supports, rather than detracts from, a peaceful death. This means hospice if you can qualify; home-based palliative care or serious illness management if you can't; and at the very minimum, prescriptions for the management of pain and anxiety. Once those basics are handled, invite a sense of calm, beauty, and focus into the room. A hospice team can help, but most of these tasks will fall to an intimate circle of friends and relatives.

Just as people in earthquake country put together kits of bottled water, dried food, and candles in anticipation of the next big one, you can create a "death kit" like those used by some hospices. The basic checklist includes a hospital bed, wheelchair, bedside commode, paper towels, dark cotton towels, diapers, and garbage bags. A "bath board," placed athwart the rim of a tub, can help you rinse or bathe a weak person if they can still be moved. Dying can be smelly, and hospice workers often bring a lavender or eucalyptus spritzer, a bag of charcoal briquettes to place under the bed to absorb odors, or a spray bottle of scentless Febreze, an effective odor-remover.

Friends can stock the kitchen with easy food and takeout menus. Bring in magazines, crossword puzzles, music, and books of poetry or religious texts—they come in handy for the long hours of waiting. Arrange a whiteboard or a notebook for people to leave each other messages.

Post documents detailing end-of-life medical wishes on the refrigerator, and make sure friends, family, and the medical team understand them. This is not something to improvise in the heat of the moment. The most helpful documents, all discussed in detail in Chapter 5, are a do-not-resuscitate order, or DNR; a POLST or MOLST, or Physician or Medical Orders for Life-Sustaining Treatment; and either a metal DNR bracelet from the Medic Alert Foundation or a plastic hospital-type DNR bracelet recognized in your particular state.

Watching someone die can be frightening, and caregivers sometimes panic and call 911. In many states, this can result in a traumatic death, or death in a hospital, because it will bring paramedics who are trained to start resuscitation first and look for paperwork later. (Saving lives—and brains—is their primary duty, and every second counts.) Therefore, make sure you have an agreed-upon alternative to calling 911. If a hospice is involved, its number should be posted by the phone. If a hospice isn't involved, I still recommend you call one immediately if death seems imminent (the person has stopped eating and drinking, for instance, or become unconscious, or extremities are turning blue) and you confront a situation you don't know how to handle. Don't give up, even if you were rejected earlier, or the dying person refused hospice services. (In Oregon, for example, some hospices can admit patients with only a few hours' notice.) Post the phone number of a primary care doctor or nurse, a physician house call service, or a clearheaded friend, preferably someone experienced with medicine or with dying, who will come over, provide reassurance, wait with you, or guide you on the phone.

PREPARING IN A NURSING HOME

Nearly a quarter of us will die in a nursing home or similar facility—often, in a shared room with someone in the next bed. There, the most important unmet need may be for privacy, not only for the vigiling family but for the roommate behind a flimsy curtain who must endure the sights, sounds and smells of death and grief.

If someone you love is dying in a nursing home, ask for a temporary private room. (You may not prevail, but it never hurts to ask.) Or improvise. When Loretta Downs's mother was dying in a nursing home in Chicago in 2006, Loretta got permission to transform an unused storage room into a sacred, private space, which she decorated with her mother's possessions. Friends and family came to share their memories and bring food, and other residents dropped in to say goodbye.

Loretta, an experienced hospice volunteer with a professional background in interior design, named the space she'd created the "Chrysalis Room" after the pupa that holds a caterpillar as it is transformed into a butterfly. The room became a permanent and beloved feature of the nursing home and set in motion a cultural shift.

Before the room was arranged, nursing home staff feared death—and the crowded conditions in which it was taking place— and sent most dying residents to the hospital. Only a few died in the nursing home under hospice care, and their families were forced to keep vigil in a room barely big enough to allow one relative to sit comfortably at the bedside. As soon as the resident died, the room would be emptied and the body taken away. The person would silently disappear from the community they'd long called home, as if they had never lived.

After the Chrysalis room opened, more residents enrolled in hospice care prior to death, and more died in the place that had become their "home," rather than in a hospital. Other residents became more likely to participate in the final goodbyes, and some became less fearful of their own deaths. Downs has since helped create similar Chrysalis rooms in nursing homes in Wyoming, Indiana, and the Chicago suburbs. The ideal spaces, she says, are quiet, with natural light, a view of nature, floor lamps, an adjustable bed, a recliner, soft music, and folding chairs. But with a little imagination, almost any private space can be made more humane than a shared room. For more information on how to improvise or build a Chrysalis room, consult Downs's endoflife inspirations.com.

GIVING CARE

Keep the dying person clean and comfortable. Turn them from side to side every two to four hours to prevent bedsores, and give adequate pain medication beforehand. This is difficult work: just do your best. Hospice nurse Jerry Soucy recommends taking your cues from the dying person: "If someone looks comfortable, they probably are, and whatever you're doing seems to be working so keep doing it," he said. "If someone looks uncomfortable, they probably are, and whatever you're doing doesn't seem to be working, so don't keep doing it."

Remember, you are watching a natural process: stopping eating and drinking is an expected part of the body shutting down, and it reduces pain and distress. Instead of coaxing or forcing food and drink, offer lip balm, Vaseline, ice chips, or a sponge soaked in water to moisten the mouth and lips.

You can relieve "air hunger" or breathlessness by opening a window, running a humidifier, or directing a small fan toward the dying person. Hospice may provide supplementary oxygen, delivered through a tube placed over the nose, but the tube can be irritating and the machine makes noise. Let comfort be your guide. If the dying person removes the tube, let it be. Worry not. Giving oxygen is unlikely to prolong dying and stopping it is unlikely to hasten it. The antianxiety drug Ativan (lorazepam), and morphine, are usually given to soothe breathlessness.

If pain and agitation don't respond, a hospice team may suggest terminal or total sedation, which creates a state of continuous unconsciousness until death comes. This sometimes requires moving the patient to a residential hospice or to a hospital, if family members are overwhelmed.

There is no right way to die. Dying people may be angry or irritable, afraid or worried, sad or accepting, or any of the above at different times. They may fear losing control, being a burden, looking undignified, or running out of money. They may want to talk about how their favorite sports teams are doing or harshly reject any talk of worldly things. They may say "I'm dying," or insist that they're going to "beat this disease" until their last breath. Some need to let go of secrets, such as having given up a child for adoption, or having been the victim or perpetrator of abuse. Some may need to hear that you will be okay without them, or that you will take care of things, or people, after they're gone. Some take their last breaths only when relatives step out of the room. So take a break once in a while.

Hearing is said to be the last sense to go. Hospice workers suggest you assume that dying people can hear everything you're saying, even after they stop responding. You may want to recall meaningful times you've had together, or qualities in them that you love. You may need to ask for forgiveness, or to thank them. Or you may feel most comfortable holding a hand in silence.

———

The ceremonies of death are for everyone present, not only the dying. Consider setting up an informal altar or table with flowers, photographs, music and candles, and, if you wish, religious images. Bring in beauty. Consider the senses: sight, touch, smell, and sound. In some areas, local branches of The Threshold Choir, a national organization, will send a small group of volunteers to sing at the bedside of any gravely ill person who asks. On the other hand, your friend may prefer listening to Willie Nelson singing "On the Road Again" through headphones. Trust the lifetime tastes of the dying person.

Soothing music, gentle touch, massaging with oil, and reading poetry or reassuring religious texts such as the 23rd Psalm (The Lord Is My Shepherd) can also help as long as they fit the dying person's tastes and beliefs. Both dying people and their attendants sometimes find the Buddhist "Metta" (Lovingkindness) prayer calming:

> May you be peaceful and at ease
> May you be filled with lovingkindness
> May you be safe, and free from fear
> May you be happy.

THE FINAL HOURS

When dying is hours away, people often pluck at sheets or blankets, reach for the light, or seem to be climbing an imaginary ladder. Their feet, fingernail beds, and lips look mottled and feel cool to the touch. Their blood pressure falls, if it's being taken, which it need not be. Their pulses may be fast, irregular, or slow.

The dying often curl into a fetal position or lie unmoving, mouth open. They lose control of their bowels and bladders. Sometimes they have convulsions and display an agitated moving-around in bed. The "death rattle" may be heard as they lose the ability to swallow and secretions build up in the throat, creating a gurgle similar to that of a leaky swimmer's snorkel. Hospice workers say it sounds worse to observers than it feels, and the secretions can be dried with eye drops containing atropine, squirted under the tongue.

Finally, most dying people stop speaking, lose consciousness, seem to be sleeping, and drift off. Breathing becomes ragged, shallow, and uneven, with long pauses between breaths, until it stops.

After death, take at least two hours before involving the world. If an expected death takes place without hospice, you might choose to first take the dog for a walk, and to say your goodbyes in ways that have meaning for you.

Make a note of the time of death, but only after you complete your goodbyes do I suggest that you notify authorities. To confirm that death has indeed taken place, you can check for a heartbeat with a stethoscope; hold a mirror up to the mouth to make sure breath does not fog it; or shine a light into the pupils of the eye to make sure they don't contract. A doctor or nurse must, by law, come to the house that day to sign the death certificate. If hospice is involved, one of its nurses can do this.

If no medical person can be found, call the business line (not the emergency line) of the county medical examiner or coroner. Make sure you tell everyone you speak with that the person had a terminal illness and has been dead for hours, and that this was an "expected death." This important term of art will minimize the chances of your home, tragic and excessive as it sounds, being regarded as a potential crime scene. Once again, try to avoid calling 911. Doing so is likely to set in motion a chain of circumstances that work against a peaceful goodbye, sometimes including forced attempts at resuscitation even if more than an hour has passed since your loved one's final breath.

HUMANIZING A HOSPITAL DEATH

Most people don't want to die in a hospital, but many do, thanks to bad luck, a sudden catastrophic turn for the worse, or a lack of realism, planning, or practical support. No matter how unexpected the situation, people *do* find ways to humanize hospital deaths and create at least some sense of a rite of passage.

We are still a long way from the day when every hospital has "dying rooms" as calm, pretty, and homey as their "birthing rooms." But even under the most unpromising circumstances, it is possible to rearrange a hospital environment to better meet the emotional and spiritual needs of the dying and those who love them.

In the spring of 2016, Liz Salmi rushed to the hospital after hearing that her beloved writing mentor Barry was on a ventilator in an intensive care unit, unable to respond in any way. He'd had a stroke, compounded by sepsis. There was no chance he'd be restored to health, little chance he'd live long, and even less chance that he'd ever again breathe on his own. His room was windowless, dark, and, as Liz wrote on her blog, "noisy with hisses, bleeps and bloops from machines . . . Everything in me screamed: *This sucks. I wouldn't want to die like this!*"

Barry had been struggling with a degenerative nerve disease for years and had signed documents indicating he didn't want to die on machines. But Barry's longtime girlfriend, his chosen advocate, was too paralyzed with shock and grief to assent to the removal of life support.

Liz and some other friends circled his bed and drew his girlfriend in while they brainstormed about how Barry might want to die. They decided on fresh air, sunlight, being outdoors, music, and dancing. One friend slipped down to her car for speakers to hook up to Barry's iPod. Another scrolled through his playlists. A third asked an ICU nurse if Barry could be wheeled outside on a gurney or in a wheelchair, so that he could die in the hospital courtyard. But the nurse said that wasn't practical.

Barry's girlfriend then asked a nurse if Barry could at least be moved to a room with natural light. The nurse nodded: the "best room" in the ICU suite was just about to open up—a sunny spot, with windows opening to the outdoors. With the assent of his girlfriend, a doctor injected Barry with sedation and after a pause, removed his breathing tube. Nurses disconnected all lines and monitors except one tracing his heartbeat. Quickly, orderlies rolled his bed into the new room.

As soon as the medical team cleared out, Liz and her friends poured in. Someone opened the windows to let in the breeze. Music played out of the little speakers. Barry's friends circled his bed, placing their hands on his legs, hands, and feet.

"Unburdened by machines," Liz wrote, "his body began sinking into the bed. As the body shifted and settled, I said, 'This is natural,' mostly to remind myself that what I was witnessing was part of the cycle of life, much like a baby crying when born." On the last functioning monitor, the bright blue line tracing Barry's heartbeat became slow and jagged.

The monitor began to ding. Someone pushed a button, silencing it. Liz held Barry's feet. "We listened through the end of the song, with our faces on Barry's, tears pouring out of our eyes," she said. "I was sobbing. We were devastated. No one danced. When the song ended, there was silence.

"A doctor wearing a white coat walked into the room. He donned a stethoscope and raised the end to Barry's chest. His hand moved to various areas of our friend's chest, and down and around to his stomach. He raised each of Barry's eyelids to shine a flashlight into the pupils, looking to see if they would constrict. The pupils did not move. The doctor looked at the clock and said, 'It is 6:11. Take as long as you need.' He exited the room. We all stood looking at Barry for a long time."

IMPROVISING RITES OF PASSAGE

To make a hospital death more sacred, beautiful, and peaceful, some family members and sympathetic nurses arrange for the removal of all telemetry and medical equipment, and the deactivation of all monitors and beeping sound effects. All of it is now unnecessary. At Kaiser Permanente hospital's emergency room in Terra Linda, California, staff follows a checklist, created by Dr. Scott Schmidt and known as the RESPECT protocol. All blood draws, diagnostic tests, and taking of vital signs are halted. Medical treatment is limited to pain management. A sign is put on the outside of the patient's door, so that staff doesn't disturb the family. Nurses are encouraged to make sure that there's a seat in the room for every family member, and that everyone is warm and comfortable.

Many hospitals, however, don't have such humane checklists. It will be up to family and friends to ask, and to otherwise reclaim the space for themselves. Some people sprinkle water around the room for a ritual cleansing. Others bring in photographs, flowers, holy books or religious icons. Even flameless electric candles can create a sacred feeling. Others get into bed with the dying person, or, with the connivance of sympathetic nurses, smuggle in the family pet (sometimes it's better to ask for forgiveness rather than permission).

In a hospital or nursing home, request a private room, and enough time to say your goodbyes and have family members present. If there's time, ask for a transfer to the hospice or palliative care service; many hospitals have them in-house. Megory Anderson, a theologian who attends the dying, often hangs sheets to create privacy if there is a roommate.

Many people, even the nonreligious, are helped by some symbolic form of letting go. In her book *Sacred Dying*, Megory describes meeting privately in a hospital with an eleven-year-old girl named Katy, who was dying of cancer and was sure God was angry with her "because of the bad things I did." It turned out she felt guilty for being mean to her brother, for being mad at her father, and especially for getting cancer, exhausting the family's money on treatments, and not getting better.

Megory took a clean sheet and tied a knot in it to represent each of the little girl's guilts. Then she and Katy called her parents and brother into the hospital room. Katy pointed to each knot and apologized for the perceived shortcoming it represented. After she completed her litany, her mother gasped and took her daughter in her arms, and Megory pulled back while the family cried and held each other. When everybody was cried out, Megory walked back to the bed, and together the family prayed and undid the knots one by one. The little girl died that night.

Others may find release from entrusting the one they love to the universe, or to otherwise saying "good journey" to what Shakespeare called "that undiscovered country from whose bourn no traveler returns." Even though my father had not been inside a church for decades except for a wedding or a funeral, I gained great comfort from a volunteer Episcopalian chaplain who anointed his head with oil and followed the "Ministration at the Time of Death" from The Book of Common Prayer.

That small ceremony, in a hospital's inpatient hospice unit, helped me acknowledge that I was turning my father over to the vast mystery from whence we come. His suffering was nearly over. It didn't matter that the precise words, about him joining "the company of the saints," no longer fit my beliefs, or his. The rite helped me say goodbye, and to acknowledge that I had come to the end of my role as my father's daughter and caregiver. I felt relieved and blessed. I do not know what comes after death, but the ceremony helped me to trust that whatever greeted my father would be benign. The time had come to stop trying to rearrange externals and to simply be present with my father for the mystery about to enter the room.

Hospice nurse Judith Redwing Keyssar, author of *Last Acts of Kindness*, remembers a beautiful young woman days away from dying of ovarian cancer in a hospital. She began moaning, "Take me home, I want to go home." Her father and brother, who'd flown in, took her literally and decided to try to move her to a hospice near Boston, where she'd grown up. While her mother spent hours holding her dying daughter's hand, the father and brother were on their cell phones, calling hospices, ambulances, and airlines. They were still making phone calls on the morning that Lily took her last breath. They'd spent her last hours in manufactured busyness.

At a certain point, let go. Sometimes a hospital team will refuse to stop treatment, and sometimes family members will disagree with each other. Accept the things you cannot change. Act in a way that will leave you with the fewest regrets, and allow the one you love to die in peace. "Come back to what is truly important," counsels hospice nurse Lori Perrine. "Pray. Reach out for guidance. Is it more important for this person to die at home, or to have a peaceful death? Sometimes they are not the same."

WELCOMING MYSTERY

It was late at night when Ed, who was teaching a photography class in Boulder, got the call. His mother, Florence, who was in her late sixties and had been in a wheelchair since suffering a stroke a year earlier, had been taken to an intensive care unit after collapsing at her front door. Paramedics had performed CPR in the driveway, despite Florence's do-not-resuscitate order. Before they succeeded in shocking her heart back into beating reliably, her brain had been deprived of oxygen for more than four minutes.

Ed drove straight from his photography class to his mother's bedside in the intensive care unit. Her hand was warm. Her body was unmoving. Her eyes were open, the pupils fixed and dilated. Her heart was still beating strongly with the help of stimulating drugs, and her lungs were filling and emptying rhythmically in time to the hush and swoosh of a mechanical ventilator.

Ed met with a critical care doctor who was blunt, brisk, and in Ed's view, callous. Florence, he said, would never think or speak again. "All of our family signed off on removing the equipment," Ed said. "It wasn't a hard decision to make."

While Ed waited in an outer room, a doctor pulled the breathing tube from Florence's throat and removed all lines, tubes, and tethers. Ed returned to the now-quiet room and took his mother's hand. Drugs were still coursing through her bloodstream, and Florence's heart kept beating and her chest kept rising and falling for more than an hour. Esther, her trusted longtime professional caregiver, sat on the other side of the bed.

As they sat their vigil, Esther talked to Ed about his mother's final weekend. Florence had been a nationally ranked championship bridge player, and she and Esther had just returned from a regional tournament in Las Vegas. The trip, which Florence had planned and executed with an unusual burst of energy and ambition, had been totally out of character with her passive, homebound life since her first stroke. With Esther at the side of her wheelchair, she'd played in almost all the available tournament games. Then they'd flown back to Denver, and Florence had collapsed before they'd even entered her house.

"This angel of a woman kept talking about how bright my mother was, and how mentally clear and lucid, and how much fun she'd had in Las Vegas," Ed said. "My mom had come in second in one [bridge] event and third in another. She'd played morning, afternoon, and evening. She had more stamina than anyone expected. It was what she loved to do, and she excelled at. She was in her joy.

"There in that ICU, I felt the overwhelming sense of a larger spirit being released from the sufferings of the body. I can't tell you specifically where it came from. It could have been all my emotion welling up for my mother. It could have been Esther, who has had a long career as a compassionate care person. But it felt larger than that.

"That tangible presence in the room with us felt larger than any experience I'd had of my mother in a physical body. It felt expansive and endless and loving and compassionate. If there was a message, despite all of these horrendous circumstances and all these machines, it was this: there was something larger there. The room was filled with love and grace."

Florence's lungs let out a long breath and did not refill. Ed thought it was the end and looked away. But Esther knew better. "There was one last breath," Ed remembered. "I didn't think it was coming, and then there was one more. It was special beyond words."

SAYING GOODBYE

In many cultures and religions, it is traditional for relatives and friends to ritually wash the body, or anoint it with oil, after death. Nurses are now bringing a beautiful nondenominational version of this ancient ceremony into hospital rooms. In 2011, Debra Rodgers, Debbie Roth, and Beth Calmes, all then nurses on the oncology unit at Cottage Health in Santa Barbara, California, created a "bathing and honoring practice" to help families—and the nurses themselves—say goodbye.

After washing and dressing the dead in clothes from home or a clean gown, the nurses encourage relatives and friends to anoint the body with lavender oil. "The physicality seems to be very helpful," said Beth Calmes. "I have a theory that after witnessing a death we go into shock, and our minds become numb and chaotic. When we start bathing and touching our loved ones, our bodies understand what our minds cannot." Here is an adapted version of their ceremony for your use.

As the hair is anointed with oil, a nurse or a family member recites, "We honor (Jane's) hair, that the wind has played with." Next a dab of oil is gently rubbed on the brow, as someone says, "We honor (Jane's) brow, the birthplace of her thoughts." In each succeeding sentence, the name of the dead person is inserted in the appropriate place.

> We honor your eyes that have looked on us with love and
> viewed the beauty of the earth.
> We honor your nostrils, the gateway of breath.
> We honor your ears that listened for our voices.
> We honor your lips that have spoken truth.
> We honor your shoulders that have borne burdens and
> strength.
> We honor your heart that has loved us.
> We honor your arms that have embraced us.
> We honor your hands that have held our hands and done so
> many things in this life.
> We honor your legs that carried you into new places of new
> challenge.
> We honor your feet that walked your own path through life.
> We give thanks to the gifts that you have given us in our life-
> time.
> We give thanks for the memories that we created together.
> We have been honored to be a part of your life.

Ways to Prepare:

At home:

- Prepare for the physical, emotional, and spiritual needs of the dying and those who love them.
- Bring in hospice if you can, and haven't already.
- Make pain management a priority.
- Plan an alternative to calling 911 in a crisis.
- Get a do-not-resuscitate order (DNR) and a POLST (Physician Orders for Life-Sustaining Treatment) or MOLST (Medical Orders for the same).
- Keep focus on what really matters: accepting whatever occurs, and having a peaceful death.

In the hospital:

- Ask for the removal of all unnecessary medical equipment, beepers, monitors, and sound effects.
- Ask for "comfort care only": no blood draws, diagnostic tests, or vital signs—only pain management.
- Don't be afraid to claim the space, smuggle in the dog, and improvise rituals that speak to you.

You may wish to recite poems or prayers. Here are some beautiful selections from around the world:

Tibetan Prayer to Be Spoken by the Dying

Through your blessing, grace, and guidance, through the power of the light that streams from you:

May all negative results from my prior actions and history, may all destructive emotions, may all obscurations, and may all blockages be purified and removed,

May I know myself forgiven for all the harm I may have thought and done,

May I accomplish this profound practice and die a good and peaceful death,

And through the triumph of my death, may I be able to
benefit all beings, living and dead.

—*Tibetan Book of the Dead*

Anglican (Episcopalian) Prayer for the Time of Death
Into your hands, O merciful Savior, we commend your servant *[insert name.]*

Acknowledge, we humbly beseech you, a sheep of your
own fold, a lamb of your own flock, a sinner of your own
redeeming.

Receive [him or her] into the arms of your mercy, into
the blessed rest of everlasting peace, and into the glorious
company of the saints in light. *Amen.*

May [his or her] soul and the souls of all the departed,
through the mercy of God, rest in peace. *Amen.*

—Book of Common Prayer

Muslim Prayer to be said by companions at the moment of death
Inna lillahi wa inna ilayhi raji'un.
Verily we belong to Allah, and truly to Him shall we return.

Hebrew Vidui (Prayer in anticipation of death)
I acknowledge before the Source of All that life and death
are not in my hands.

Just as I did not choose to be born, so I do not choose
to die.

May my life be a healing memory for those who knew me.

May my loved ones think well of me, and may my memory bring them joy.

From all those I may have hurt, I ask forgiveness.

To all who have hurt me, I grant forgiveness.

As a wave returns to the ocean, so I return to the Source
from which I came.

Toward a New Art of Dying

Fear no more the heat o' the sun

Fear no more the heat o' the sun,
Nor the furious winter's rages;
Thou thy worldly task hast done,
Home art gone, and ta'en thy wages:
Golden lads and girls all must,
As chimney sweepers come to dust.

Fear no more the frown o' the great;
Thou art past the tyrant's stroke;
Care no more to clothe and eat;
To thee the reed is as the oak:
The scepter, learning, physic, must
All follow this, and come to dust.

Fear no more the lightning flash,
Nor the all-dreaded thunder stone;
Fear not slander, censure rash;
Thou hast finished joy and moan:
All lovers young, all lovers must
Consign to thee, and come to dust.

No exorciser harm thee!
Nor no witchcraft charm thee!
Ghost unlaid forbear thee!
Nothing ill come near thee!
Quiet consummation have;
And renownèd be thy grave!

—WILLIAM SHAKESPEARE, from *Cymbeline*

EVERYTHING BROKE HER WAY

I close this book with a story of the late Louise Manfreddi, who got the care that all dying people deserve, and few get. Her "good death" was the fruit of seamless long-term collaboration among her family members, doctors, nurses, and others. She was the daughter of poor Methodist ministers in upstate New York. Her husband, Gene, was a house painter. In the 1950s, they bought a home in Syracuse, where she worked as a school aide and raised two daughters, Anne and Lee. In her spare time, she gardened, read voraciously, started a feminist consciousness-raising group, and loved to talk about politics. When she was in her mid-fifties, she suffered a crippling brain bleed and was never again capable of managing daily life on her own.

After months of despair, Louise built a new life with the help of her family. She learned to walk and talk again, partly by watching *Sesame Street*, but she never regained the capacity to sequence practical tasks. She could warm a cup of coffee in the microwave, but not make it from scratch. She could read an article, but not a book. She needed her husband or one of her daughters to lay out her clothes in the morning and to help her wash her hair. She had to stop gardening and driving, but she returned to keeping up with politics and seeing family friends. She volunteered as a greeter at her church, always wearing a maroon beret; she often sat in a pew with people who'd come alone.

She died at the age of eighty-four, of pneumonia, in a beautiful oak-paneled hospice on a hill above Syracuse, her home town. As she took her last breaths, her daughters were holding her hands. Her body smelled sweet, thanks to a compassionate orderly who (with the family's permission) had washed her and anointed her body with fragrant oils.

Many of us hope for good deaths if we fill out advance directives and get comfortable, on a spiritual level, with the reality of death in the abstract. We hope to die at home and avoid intensive care. But a good death often requires more support than the right paperwork and the right state of mind.

Louise got it. Thanks to an innovative federal program, she had the best experience of death, despite a difficult long decline, of anybody I've ever known. In her last eight years, she was in the hospital only once. She never spent a single night in a nursing home. She had the extraordinary luck to be diverted from the disjointed medical care experienced by most American elders and into an integrated program that supported her from beginning to end. She died a better death than many people I know with more money and education, and Rolodexes full of influential names.

Her pathway to a good death started, oddly enough, with a botched colonoscopy when she was seventy-six. She was taken to St. Joseph's Hospital in Syracuse for surgery to remove a perforated section of her colon. There, a perceptive social worker took a close look at her husband. Louise's daughters had long since married and moved out, and Gene, who'd retired early on Social Security to care for his increasingly dependent wife, was spent. In a tearful family meeting at the hospital, the social worker persuaded Louise to enter the Alzheimer's unit of a local nursing home.

The stay gave Gene a break. But Louise was bored, miserable, and far more mobile and alert than her fellow residents with classic Alzheimer's, some of whom spent the day weeping in their wheelchairs. She wanted to go home. But Gene couldn't manage alone anymore, and he balked at selling their house and using the money to move with her into some form of assisted living. Bringing in private health aides wasn't an option, because the Manfreddis couldn't afford them, and in any case didn't want to give up their privacy.

It was then that Louise's daughter Lee, a web designer, searched online and found an innovative federally funded program called PACE. The mission of the Program of All-Inclusive Care for the Elderly is to keep people like Louise at home, by providing extensive support to their caregivers. A program was just starting up in Syracuse, as part of Loretto, a nonprofit founded by the local Catholic diocese, that had been looking after the elderly since 1926. Loretto was closely affiliated with St. Joseph's Health, another nonprofit whose flagship hospital had been named a "best regional hospital" by *U.S. News and World Report.* The Syracuse program, like all PACE programs, was modeled on a pioneering effort, begun in 1971 in San Francisco's Chinatown, called "On Lok," which means "peaceful happy home" in Cantonese. Started by a social worker and a dentist, On Lok was never promoted as a pathway to a good death. Its goal was to keep fragile elderly people healthy, strong, and well-supported enough to stay with their families in the Chinese community, rather than being funneled into hospitals and nursing homes.

For the Manfreddis, the PACE emphasis on living a good life was the first step on the pathway to a very good death. As soon as Louise entered the program, the lives of everyone in her family changed. A nurse came to the house and made sure Gene was strong enough to keep his wife at home with adequate support, and an occupational therapist checked to see that the house itself was safe. (A PACE handyman followed later to make recommended upgrades, such as adding grab bars and railings.) A PACE social worker helped the couple fill out the paperwork to qualify Louise for Medicaid (which, along with Medicare, would pay PACE a monthly lump sum to cover Louise's care) and got the couple to prepay for funeral plans, which wouldn't be counted against them in assessing their Medicaid application.

Making burial plans flowed naturally into getting the couple thinking about the end of life. The nurse arranged for a MOLST (Medical Order for Life-Sustaining Treatment) form, signed by a PACE doctor, detailing Louise's medical wishes. She chose her husband, Gene, and her daughter Lee to make her decisions when she could no longer make her own.

From then on, PACE handled all of Louise's care in one inclusive package. It made no distinction between curative medicine, rehabilitation, social work, having fun, socializing, and practical support. It provided them all, and it saw her not as a diagnosis, but as a whole person, and it ministered to her body, heart, and soul. Three days a week, a van took Louise to a daycare program in a converted commercial building in Syracuse, giving Gene a break. From there, she and other PACE participants often set out on field trips, to view pumpkin festivals or fall leaves, and to visit casinos and movie theaters.

PACE served everyone lunch and sent Louise home with dinner and food for the weekend. In midwinter, the PACE group toured "Lights on the Lake," a set of elaborate displays of Christmas lights arrayed around Onondaga Lake. Louise was beloved by PACE attendants, who saw their work as a calling, not a job. The van drivers and home health aides were crucial members of the PACE team, and they were often the first to notice signs of health problems in clients. Their observations helped nip issues in the bud, and they were included in the regular case conferences held to discuss each client.

When Louise developed cataracts, she got surgery. When she was diagnosed with macular degeneration, a PACE van drove her to an ophthalmologist for expensive injections to slow its progress. PACE paid for hearing aids, because hearing well keeps people social, and happily social people are less likely to have their dementias worsen. It covered eyeglasses and dentures, unlike standard Medicare. She could get her hair done for ten dollars at a beauty shop at the daycare program, enjoy visiting musicians and pets, and see a podiatrist and a physical therapist, too—all at no charge to the family. Once a week, a PACE attendant came to the house to help her bathe. A nurse was on call twenty-four hours a day, and when Louise got sick, one came to the house.

PACE paid for an alert device in case she fell. It sent her home with plastic-wrapped packets of her medications, labeled by day, hour, and dose, so that all her husband had to do was rip the packages open and give them to her at the right times. When she became incontinent, PACE delivered the right-size diapers. "What that meant was that my mother could live with my dad, who had no special training," said her daughter Lee. "He could concentrate on being her husband and keeping the house together."

In her last year of life, Louise stopped being a greeter at her church and grew increasingly weak and quiet. She lost ten pounds without intending to. Nobody talked about her dying, but it was evident that she was in steep decline. She grew gently delusional, congratulating one daughter for a nonexistent work promotion, and consoling the other about an imaginary financial crisis that was supposedly forcing her to sell her house and to move away. She went to the daycare center less and napped for hours on the couch at home. She lost the ability to swallow vigorously enough to prevent food from entering her lungs, and she endured a bout of pneumonia, which was treated with antibiotics at home.

After she recovered, PACE attendants came to the house three times a day to puree food for her. A nutritionist went to great lengths to stimulate her appetite, and everyone turned a blind eye to the fact that Gene also fed her ice cream. It was a tacit trade-off: to allow her simple pleasures rather than turning what remained of her life into a grim death-postponing project.

Shortly before Thanksgiving in 2015, Gene woke up in terror in the middle of the night. Louise was lying next to him, struggling to breathe, making horrible, rattling sounds. He called an ambulance. Louise had again contracted pneumonia.

At St. Joseph's Hospital, which cared for all PACE clients, it was touch and go. When they first arrived, Gene wasn't sure his wife would make it through the next ten minutes. Nurses set up a thin tube at her nostrils to deliver high-flow oxygen, and inserted intravenous lines for antibiotics to fight the infection, and saline to counter dehydration. Louise rallied at first and stopped panting for breath. But she didn't get better; in fact, each day she got worse. Fluid was building up in the space between her lungs and the chest wall.

About a week after her arrival, her doctors asked her and her family whether they'd agree to a thoracentesis, in which a long, thick needle would be inserted between Louise's ribs to draw out the fluid and make it easier for her to breathe. It would probably make Louise feel better temporarily, the doctors said. But the procedure itself would be painful, it wouldn't permanently cure the problem, and it carried risks of its own. As Lee remembers it, "My sister Anne asked the doctors, 'If it was your mom or your sister, would you do it?' They [the doctors] danced around it with their words, but with their eyes and their faces, they said 'no.'"

Louise curiously insisted she didn't have pneumonia and that the fluid wasn't bothering her, so Anne told the doctors, "Let's not do it." She and Lee were guided in part by conversations the family had had around the kitchen table years earlier, expressing sadness over a beloved relative who'd developed dementia and spent years curled up on a feeding tube in a nursing home. They were also helped by the fact that eight years earlier, Louise had expressed her medical preferences when she entered the PACE program. "When in the hospital, it became apparent that this was not going anywhere good," Lee remembers. "The MOLST gave us exactly the guidance we would have wanted."

At this point, a medical team with a different philosophy, in a less well-coordinated and more financially driven medical system might have persuaded Louise to submit to the procedure to withdraw fluid. There'd have been good reimbursement for it and the day of reckoning could have been postponed. If the family had resisted, a doctor might have made dire predictions about how she would suffer and die. Doctors could have tried ever more exotic and expensive antibiotics, and powerful drugs to get her blood pressure down. If she'd been a nursing home resident without family to protect her, she might have ended up in intensive care, and died there.

This didn't happen.

Ten days after entering the hospital, Louise started saying she wasn't hungry or thirsty; she refused food and water and grew less responsive. She still was on an intravenous saline drip and antibiotics, comfortable, conscious, and not in pain. Thanksgiving came, and after Lee returned from celebrating with her in-laws, a social worker from PACE convened a big family meeting around Louise's bed. Her husband, Gene, sat in a plastic chair at its foot with his head in his hands. Lee sat on one side of her mother, her sister Anne on the other. Standing near the head of the bed were a young doctor-in-training, his physician supervisor from the hospital's palliative care team, two social workers (one from the hospital, one from PACE), and a nurse. They were all there to discuss what doctors call "goals of care."

Her daughter Lee doesn't remember the words the young doctor used as he made his first fumbling attempt. His supervising doctor stepped in and gave it another try. But nothing they said registered with Gene, who just sat there with his head in his hands. "They were talking medical," Lee remembers. "They were saying things like 'We are concerned about her care,' and 'we want to keep her comfortable.' They just danced around it. They were more uncomfortable than we were! They were saying we could move her into a nursing home, and giving a whole laundry list of options as if she was going to live another five months.

"Finally, I got exasperated. I grabbed Dad's hands and said, 'Let me see if I can summarize. What these kind people are too kind to say out loud is that we're discussing what kind of death we're going to give Mom.'"

Everyone exhaled. "The elephant in the room was acknowledged," Lee said, "and everyone was free to be more specific." The doctors asked whether the family would agree to take Louise off antibiotics and stop the intravenous saline drip keeping her hydrated. It would make her more comfortable not to be tethered, and it would allow her to die a little sooner and easier. Perhaps the family would like to think about it overnight.

Neither Gene, nor his daughters, felt pressured or even nudged. "If we'd said we wanted them to pull out all the stops [and give maximum treatment] they would have done it," Lee said. "We were given the time and the opportunity to make our own decisions." With tears running down his face, Louise's husband looked up. "What's the point?" he said. Louise he knew, had always wanted to die before he did. In fact, she'd often joked that if he dared to die first, she'd kill him. "She always wanted to go first," Gene said. "Let's give her that. Let's do it now, take her off the antibiotics."

Now Lee assumed the role of the family's chief negotiator. If they said yes to palliative care, she asked the medical team, what were her mother's options? Classic hospice wasn't an option unless Louise disenrolled from PACE, and signed up for hospice, which she wouldn't live long enough to do. In any case, her daughters didn't think that they, as a family, could make their mother as comfortable as a skilled nursing staff could. "We wanted our job to be present with her as family and not be her care staff," Lee remembers. "We didn't think having her die at home would be in our father's best interests. We couldn't imagine that he would ever want to sleep in that bed again."

At that point, the PACE social worker suggested "a wonderful ward on the top floor" of The Cunningham, a high-rise nursing home, and a beautifully integrated part of Loretto's care system. Cunningham had adopted an acclaimed innovation in nursing home culture called the Eden Alternative, which eliminates industrialized, division-of-labor approaches to nursing home care, and clusters residents instead in small groups where they can build deeper relationships with a few staff members, and with each other. PACE would cover Louise's bills there, just as they had at St. Joseph's. And thanks to a federal grant of more than a million dollars, the top floor of Cunningham had been turned into a beautiful, long-term palliative care, nursing, and hospice unit. Lee pressed the hospital staff hard: if they agreed to let Louise leave the hospital, would the team guarantee that Louise got a bed on the top floor of Cunningham? The PACE social worker paused and said she would do her best.

From then on, things moved rapidly. The hospital's discharge planning department sprang into action, pressing to serve the institutional goal of freeing up Louise's bed. Only a few beds on the top floor of Cunningham were earmarked for dying patients, and at that hour none was empty. The discharge planner decided to send Louise to an open bed on another nursing floor of Cunningham, one with none of the palliative floor's amenities. Louise could move to the top floor, the discharge planner said, as soon as a bed opened up. The ever savvy and vigilant Lee objected. She immediately called Medicare and filed an appeal against the "discharge plan." The appeals process automatically bought Louise an extra day in the hospital, and during that time, someone died on the top floor of Cunningham. To the relief of her family, Louise was moved there by medical transport van.

Dying can be ugly, and families and friends thirst for beauty. A good death is judged not only by the peace and comfort of the dying person, but by the memories that inhabit, or later haunt, those who survive it. Lee vividly remembers the Cunningham's oak paneling and its expansive views of the valley. The husbands, sisters, children, and wives of the dying weren't huddled around a vending machine drinking bad coffee and anticipating worse news. Instead they gathered around a fireplace in the living room, prepared meals in a common kitchen, and ate family-style in a dining room around a long Mission Oak refectory table. The attendants weren't called "certified nursing assistants," but *anam cara*, which means "soul friend" in Gaelic. They were encouraged to focus on nurturing their relationships with residents, not on punching out a list of tasks. The walls, the paneling, the furniture, the kitchen, everything said: you are not a patient. Those who love you are not visitors. Your dying is a human, not a medical, event. You and those you love will be cared for, and you will die in beauty.

In this institution, funded by the government, medicine was fulfilling its last forgotten duty: to attend the dying. Louise's room was as big as a luxury hotel room, spacious enough to hold two cots, and there Lee and her sister Anne slept during the four days it took their mother to die. In the daytime, they would wheel their mother's bed over to the window and sit on either side of her for hours, each holding one of her hands. The sisters could take a breath and look out at the clouds, hills, lakes, and valleys that surround Syracuse. They heard not the beeping of cardiac monitors, but music Louise loved—recordings of strings, flutes, and Christmas music that Anne played on a boom box that her sister Lee borrowed from staff on the thirteenth floor.

Each day, staff members brought the sisters food, so they only left their mother's side when they needed to step outside for some fresh air. Every two hours, attendants—the *anam caras*—came in to gently wash and turn Louise so she was kept clean and comfortable, and her skin didn't break down.

Louise didn't look beautiful. She'd lost some weight in her final year, more in the hospital, and even more since she'd stopped eating and drinking. Her skull showed through her skin. Strands of her thin gray hair were plastered to her head. A plastic oxygen tube trailed from her nostrils to soothe air hunger. She was incontinent. Her body was skeletal. She sunk into herself and said less and less. But there was a pink quilt on the bed and her hand was curled around a pillow, embroidered with a heart, brought in by her daughter Anne. The emotional and spiritual needs of the family remained at the center of things, and frantic medical attempts to ignore or forestall death had no place.

Louise had always believed in a loving God, but she'd never placed much stock in the notion of hell. "Do you think there's a heaven?" she'd often asked her daughter Lee. "I don't think there are fluffy clouds," Lee had said. "But the energy is never lost." When Louise was near death, Lee asked her mother if she was afraid of dying. "You could see her gathering all her resources and pulling herself up to consciousness. She said 'no.'"

On the morning of the fourth day, Louise's hands and feet turned a dusky blue. Her breathing grew slow and ragged. After washing her and cleaning her bed, one of Cunningham's attendants, a man named Cesar who'd been born in Puerto Rico, asked her daughters, "Is it okay with you if I pray for your mom?" After they said yes and stepped aside briefly, Cesar anointed Louise's head and body with fragrant oils and conducted a small service, reading to her softly from his Spanish Bible.

A few hours after Cesar finished, Lee saw that Louise's breaths were coming farther and farther apart. She took her dying mother's hand again and told her, as her sister had earlier, that she'd been a good Mom and it was okay to go. Lee held a phone up to Louise's ear. Louise's husband, Gene, who'd found it too painful to be at her side for more than a few hours a day, was at home, too far away to make it back in time. He told his wife again how much he loved her. Hearing Gene's voice, Louise took her final breath. She was eighty-four.

Lee took out a vial of colored consecrated sand that had been given to her by Tibetan monks during a mandala ceremony at a nearby Native American cultural center. She sprinkled a few grains on her mother's body. She took off her mother's wedding rings and put them in her pocket.

It had been cloudy all that day. Outside the window, a hole in the clouds broke open and the sun came streaming through. Then the opening slowly filled with clouds again. This came, for the Manfreddi sisters, at exactly the right time. "We felt that was how and when our mother finally left her body," Lee said. "That was when heaven, the universal consciousness, or whatever you believe comes next, opened to embrace her."

Fifteen minutes later, a nurse came into the room. She listened for a heartbeat, confirmed to the sisters that their mother was dead, and accepted their report of the time of death without intrusion, drama, or bustle. "It was empowering because our word wasn't challenged, and we weren't berated for not calling in an "authority," Lee remembers. "It made her death and our vigil feel like a personal and familial rite of passage, not a legal event." The nurse let the sisters know she'd call a doctor, get the death certificate signed, and notify the funeral home. "She was gone. It was like a switch had been flipped." They kissed their mother's body goodbye, tucked the covers under her chin, and left to be with their father.

This is what a collaborative death can look like. Louise's family was neither exhausted nor broke. From the day she entered the PACE program until she took her last breath, the care she got—far broader than what we usually think of as "medicine"—had been attuned to her needs, and had never ignored what she and her family valued. With one minor exception, her family had never had to fight with a doctor, a hospital, or a government agency.

The aftertaste of her death was not bitterness or bewilderment, but gratitude. "It brings tears to my eyes to think about her passing, but they are tears of feeling the loss, not about how or why she died or anything we did or didn't do," said her daughter Lee. "She didn't have to suffer through a long nursing home residence or hospital stay. I am comforted that our family and our community could give her a good death, without pain, and almost in her own bed. We have no regrets and only hope we are privileged to make our own departures with as much grace. It was a perfect storm. Everything broke her way."

Louise's death is a model for the nation. Everyone facing the end of life should have access to this level of coordinated medical and practical, even spiritual, care. It is a travesty that our society spends so much money on futile, painful high-technology medical care near the end of life, while depriving so many of the simple supports they need to die peacefully. I wish this book could promise that you, and those you love, will pass through the difficult passages of later life as well as Louise did. But I can't. She had the good luck to live in Syracuse, which is blessed by an excellent integrated health system, started by altruistic people with something other than profit in mind. She had an assertive, diplomatic daughter with a backbone to act as her medical advocate. And finally, she had the PACE program, which places its clients, not institutional convenience, at the heart of its mission.

For many of the rest of us, our final years will probably be, at times, chaotic. PACE currently serves only forty thousand frail elders nationwide. It has friends in Congress, but it doesn't have an army of highly paid lobbyists, and it's not high enough on the national agenda to be significantly expanded. It is widely acknowledged that in most parts of the country, the conventional medical system—at least in its approach to the aging, incurably ill, and dying—is broken. You and those who love you are walking a labyrinth full of blind alleys, cracks, and broken steps. You may not be able to find a physician who makes house calls. You may not have a fierce and dedicated family member or health care advocate. You will have to navigate what the 2014 Institute of Medicine's report on Dying in America called "a fragmented delivery system, spurred by perverse financial incentives" and a tragic "mismatch between the services patients and families need and the services they can obtain." In such an environment, even a good-enough decline, and a good-enough death, is a triumph.

I have introduced you to some of the people, inside and outside medicine, who are improvising ways to make our last months, and theirs, more humane. They include street angels like the nurses who make house calls to the frail elderly in Santa Barbara, California, and the emergency room doctor in the Kaiser Permanente system who makes sure that the relatives of a dying person have places to sit, warm blankets, and the necessary privacy to say goodbye. They include a quiet army of physical therapists, occupational therapists, social workers, hospice nurses, and palliative care and geriatrics doctors who focus on keeping people functioning well and enjoying the best possible quality of life until it's time for a good quality of death. They include the thousands of informal circles of people who organize the care of a dying friend, and the millions of paid caregivers who regard their poorly compensated work as a calling. It includes the nurses who wash and honor the bodies of the dead, bringing the sacred back into the hospital room with as much dignity as did the rituals of our ancestors. I hope you will find your way to such people, and when you can't, to follow their examples and make up your own versions of what they do.

The challenge for our society is to take what are now scattered experiments, fueled mainly by philanthropies, Medicare pilot programs, and the altruism of individuals, and make them the standard of care for everyone undergoing the expected transitions of the last quarter of life. This will require a revolt from the bottom up. We deserve more, we should expect more, and the health care dollars to pay for it are already being spent, but mainly on expensive, harrowing technologies that do little lasting good. Some version of the PACE pathway, tailored to fit individual needs, should be available to every declining, incurably ill, and dying person in America. All fragile individuals should get physician house calls. Anybody who needs medical care at home should get hospice, not only those whose diseases march fast enough to predict death within six months.

To do so will require a change in the reimbursement system.

Today, the most poorly paid people in medicine are those who meet the needs of aging and incurably ill people, and are honest about the reality of death. An oncologist who spends hours with his patients, tries to understand what matters to them, explains the limits of medicine, and encourages them to explore hospice, will get poorer reviews from his patients, and make less money, than the one who never tells the truth and administers futile and grueling, but well-reimbursed, chemotherapies until days before death. A doctor who specializes in geriatrics will make less money than an internist with less training, and both will earn hundreds of thousands of dollars less per year than a cardiac surgeon or intensive care specialist. Penny-wise and pound-foolish medical insurance systems, including Medicare, continue to be stingy about funding physical therapy, which delays disability and supports continued well-being, while lavishly reimbursing $6,000 ambulance rides and $7,000-a-day intensive care units for people who fall because they didn't get physical therapy. That system needs to be turned upside down, so that it better rewards practitioners who take time and put patients at the center of concern, and rewards deploying technologies less well. As it stands now, the reimbursement system is practically engineered to produce expensive, overly medicalized deaths, full of unnecessary suffering. It takes enormous gumption, savvy, support—and luck, and sometimes money—to find the way to a peaceful passage.

Our current system is structured for the convenience of the richest and most powerful one percent of the players in medicine—hospitals, insurance companies, specialists, academic medical centers, and commercial companies that sell drugs and medical devices for profit. It does a better job of benefiting them than it does at serving the patients who supposedly lie at the heart of medicine's mission. It is time we, the silent majority who serve, or will serve, in the nation's informal Caregiver Army, found our voices on every level, starting with the individual doctor's office.

THE ART OF THE IMPERFECT

I hope this book will help you to navigate this bewildering situation wisely. I hope it will give you the tools to reverse incipient health problems while you still can; to get well-coordinated medical care when you can't reverse them; and to recruit someone to protect you from aggressive treatment when you become fragile. I hope it encourages you to never be intimidated by a doctor, to remain the expert on your own life, and to keep your voice. Above all, I hope this book will help you shape your life, and your death, in ways that reflect what matters most to you. I hope that no matter where you die, someone brave will help you make room for the sacred.

But please remember that we create a new Art of Dying not to make things perfect. We work with the inadequate materials at hand to fashion something bearable, shared, and in its own way beautiful because it is sanctified by love.

People like the physician-writer Atul Gawande are making amazing strides in improving the culture of medicine from the top down, coaching doctors to hold more honest conversations with people confronting the unfixable. But training doctors to tell patients what they need to know is only one piece of the puzzle. It's up to the rest of us, working from the bottom up, to create the political pressure to transform private and public insurance so that they financially reward such changes, and give us the practical and medical support we need near the end of life.

So find your voice. Your best conversations about aging, dying, and medicine will probably not take place in a doctor's office. They'll take place around your kitchen table, with you speaking your own kitchen table language to the people you love, and who love you. And then I urge you to take your voice out into the wider world, and keep telling your stories.

Glossary

Many professions speak a secret language, intimidating to outsiders. Medicine is no exception. It is riddled with professional jargon, acronyms, euphemisms, overly officious terms for simple concepts, slang, and secret argot. Since the subculture of medicine can be mysterious, I hope this glossary of its terms of art will be a guide, much like a phrase book for a foreign country. The aim is to empower you to understand what your doctors are trying to tell you, and encourage you to speak up about what matters most to you.

ADLs (Activities of Daily Living): A checklist of the five basic tasks required to carry on an independent daily life: feeding ourselves, bathing, dressing, grooming, and going to the toilet. They are important because assessing ADLs is a quick way to set therapeutic goals for improved functioning, and to qualify for various Medicare and Medicaid benefits. **IADLs** (instrumental activities of daily living) are the more sophisticated life tasks necessary to function well in complex modern society, such as paying bills, cleaning house, shopping, cooking, driving, taking medications on time, and using the phone. People having trouble with IADLs can often cope at home with sporadic assistance, while those having trouble with ADLs usually need help daily or even hourly.

Advance directive, or AD: Also called a living will, this legal document records the treatments you want and don't want when you are unable to communicate, close to dying, or unlikely to be restored to a life that you consider enjoyable and meaningful. If you fear being hooked up to a ventilator when you are dying, or being kept "alive" after a catastrophic brain injury, sign an advance directive.

Advanced illness: Doctor's lingo for the later stages of serious, slow-moving, incurable, and ultimately fatal conditions, such as cancer, emphysema, and heart failure. This phrase has no set medical definition and no timetable, but it generally means that you can no longer function without help, and no turnaround is in sight. Ask your doctor precisely what she means if she uses this phrase; in some cases, she may mean you are "hospice ready."

Anticholinergics: Insidious, widely used medications, ranging from Benadryl to many prescription sleeping pills, that block the action of the chemical acetylcholine in the brain and nervous system. Short-term use is linked to cognitive confusion; longer-term use is linked to a significantly higher risk of dementia. For more information, consult the "Beers List," frequently updated by the American Geriatrics Society.

Assisted suicide or physician-assisted suicide: Terms used by opponents of the practice of prescribing life-ending medications to terminally ill people who request them. Because the word "suicide" has criminal and pathological connotations, proponents prefer the terms "aid-in-dying," "right to die," "death with dignity," "physician-assisted death," and "end-of-life options."

Attending: An attending physician is the top dog among the doctors you are likely to see in a hospital. He or she trains and supervises less-experienced interns and residents. The rule of thumb is the longer the coat, the higher the doctor's status and power. Interns are the newbies in the short white jackets; residents are halfway through their training; and attendings generally wear the longest coats. If you want a change in your hospital care (such as no taking vital signs at night) ask the attending to write a **physician's order**.

Bioethics committee: A group appointed by a hospital to resolve conflicts among doctors, families, and patients about treatment (and nontreatment) by applying the basic principles of medical ethics. The four guiding principles are: patient autonomy, fairness, non-harming, and benefiting the patient. (Usually summarized as autonomy, justice, non-maleficence, and beneficence.) If you feel you are getting medical treatment you don't want, or not getting care you do want, you can ask for a "bioethics consult." A palliative care consultation, however, is usually a better first step, because palliative care doctors are often more interpersonally skilled, and negotiate practical solutions.

Capacity: Medical-legal term for having the marbles to make your own decisions. If your doctors decide you don't have "capacity," decision-making will fall to your designated medical advocate— also known as your **surrogate**, health care agent or **proxy**—and if you have none, to the doctors themselves.

Care: This term means very different things to medical staff and to lay people and creates much confusion. In the medical world, "care" means any form of treatment, including intrusive and un-comfortable life support technologies. It doesn't necessarily mean hands-on nursing, emotional support, and other forms of what lay people call "caring." When a doctor speaks of "withdrawing care," he or she usually means releasing a dying person from advanced medical technologies, not the end of concern, comfort, and com-passion for the patient.

Charge nurse: The nurse "in charge" of the shift on your hospital ward. The decision maker. If you want a change in your nursing care, don't just complain, ask for the charge nurse.

Chemo brain: Mental fog, often permanent, following chemo-therapy. One of many causes of dementia.

Chronic: Incurable but often manageable. People with well-managed chronic illnesses sometimes survive for decades.

Chronic obstructive pulmonary disease (COPD): A serious lung disease, such as emphysema, in which lungs become less efficient at delivering oxygen to your bloodstream. COPD is incurable; you will qualify for hospice when it is **advanced** or **end stage**.

Circling the drain: Doctor-to-doctor slang for "approaching the end of life," used for frail patients suffering repeated health crises. Any crisis may be the last. More scientific-sounding terms include advanced frailty, **multiple co-morbidities**, and **failure to thrive**.

Clinical effectiveness: A measure of direct benefit to a patient's well-being. It is important to ask about "clinical effectiveness," because many treatments that show "surrogate effectiveness" or "statistical significance" improve scores on diagnostic tests but don't translate into real benefits for real patients.

Coding: Hospital slang for imminently dying, also called crashing. The term comes from announcing a Code Blue over a hospital public address system, to request a resuscitation team. A *slow code*, *light blue code*, or *Hollywood code* means going through the motions of a Code Blue to satisfy relatives or hospital protocols, but doing so slowly and gently because there is no hope of saving the patient. Other codes are not standardized from hospital to hospital, but Code Red usually indicates a fire.

Comfort care: Phrase used in hospitals and nursing homes for stopping any treatment that causes pain, and focusing instead on relieving all forms of suffering. It has no precise medical definition but the term is widely recognized. If you think it's time to stop curative measures and allow a natural death, ask for a **physician's order** for "comfort care" or "comfort measures only."

Complementary and alternative medicine: All non-Western and non-traditional approaches to sickness and health are lumped together under this heading, including acupuncture, nutrition, reiki, guided imagery, massage, ayurveda, herbs, and harmonizing mind and body through prayer or meditation. An umbrella term for healing modalities developed outside the western scientific paradigm.

Congestive heart failure (CHF): The heart no longer pumps efficiently, due to leaky valves, stiff and clogged vessels, or other damage. A chronic, incurable, worsening condition. Symptoms include breathlessness, fatigue, weakness, and swollen ankles. Sometimes a pacemaker, a heart valve replacement, or another surgery can help if the patient is still resilient. Often symptoms are best managed with medications and lifestyle changes such as exercising, reducing salt, managing stress, and losing weight. In its early stages, a heart management nurse can help you maintain the best possible quality of life. CHF usually worsens until it becomes **advanced** or **end stage**, making it a hospice-qualifying diagnosis. Hospice nurses can help you manage shortness of breath, heart pain, and other symptoms, using morphine and other drugs.

Cowboy: A medical risk taker. This disparaging in-house term is used to describe doctors who take inappropriate risks, such as performing open-heart surgery on someone too weak to recover. If you get news you don't like from one doctor, you can probably find a "cowboy" willing to blue-sky you.

CPR: An attempt at reviving a person after stoppage of the heart or breathing, using stimulating drugs, forceful pushes on the chest, and shocking of the heart with an external defibrillator. When performed on the frail elderly or the terminally ill, CPR can break ribs and be brutal and ineffective. Short-term survival rates range from 8 to 20 percent, and survival without brain damage is rare. To avoid CPR, get a physician to sign a **POLST** and/ or a **do-not-resuscitate (DNR)** or **allow natural death (AND)** order.

Crash cart: Rolling hospital cart containing drugs and devices for cardiopulmonary resuscitation (CPR), including a hand-operated airbag mask to support breathing, and an external defibrillator to attempt to shock the heart back into a normal rhythm.

Cyanosis: Being blue. Blue lips, skin, and fingernail beds are common signs of the approach of death.

Defibrillator: An external defibrillator shocks the heart through the chest wall in an attempt to normalize its rhythm. An implanted defibrillator, or ICD, sometimes called "an emergency room in your chest," does the same thing internally. When it fires, people say it feels like "being kicked in the chest by a horse." If you agree to a defibrillator, it is important to create an "exit plan" for a deactivation order when it no longer serves your purposes, as it can cause unnecessary suffering and repeated painful shocks on the deathbed. According to joint ethical statements issued by all the major cardiology associations, deactivation is neither assisted suicide nor euthanasia.

Dementia: Practical medical shorthand for a decrease in mental function severe enough to require help managing daily life. Because it has multiple causes, dementia is a label, not a precise diagnosis.

Do Not Hospitalize (DNH) or Do Not Transport (DNT): Physicians' orders to prohibit you from being transported to a hospital, so that you can die in the place that has become your home. This order is often part of a **POLST**.

Do-not-resuscitate (DNR) or allow natural death (AND) order: A doctor's order forbidding cardiopulmonary resuscitation; it is difficult to get a doctor to write a DNR unless you have a terminal illness.

Dying: A word many doctors avoid, instead preferring to say *multiple organ systems failure, advanced, or end stage.*

Edema: Swelling from retained fluid.

Emesis: Vomiting

End stage: Medical language for approaching the end of life, usually due to a slowly moving disease, such as congestive heart failure, emphysema, or kidney failure. The term has no precise medical meaning, but when doctors use it, they usually think death is likely within six months. If your doctor uses this phrase, ask him or her to explain in more detail what he or she means, and ask about hospice. You will probably qualify and do considerably better with its services.

End stage renal disease (ESRD): Kidney failure, in which the kidneys lose the ability to filter toxins from the blood. Without dialysis or a kidney transplant, ESRD leads, usually within months, to a relatively painless death, marked by fatigue, mental confusion, and a gradual slipping into unconsciousness.

Euthanasia: Mercy killing. From the Greek, meaning "a good death." It is now used to mean having one's life ended *involuntarily* by medical means, which is illegal. The term is also sometimes inaccurately used to describe the *voluntary* timing of one's own death with prescribed medications, which is legal for the terminally ill in several states and is better known as aid-in-dying or physician-assisted death.

Evidence-based medicine (EBM): Making clinical decisions on the basis of scientific evidence that a treatment is effective. At its best, EBM leads to abandoning ineffective treatments and making medical care more consistent in large health systems; at its worst, it devolves into cookie-cutter medicine done by algorithm rather than by developing a healing relationship between doctor and patient.

Failure to thrive: An official catchall medical diagnosis overlapping with "the dwindles" and advanced frailty, characterized by a weight loss of more than 5 percent, poor appetite, weakness, and low energy. When not caused by dehydration, depression, or another correctable cause, failure to thrive is often a harbinger of the final decline. On its own, it is no longer a hospice-qualifying diagnosis. Privately, doctors sometimes use **circling the drain**.

Fatal: Another word doctors don't like to use, instead preferring terminal, progressive, serious, chronic, or end-stage.

Feeding tubes or PEG tubes: Delivery of nutrition via a tube through the nose or implanted directly in the stomach. Nursing homes find them convenient and well-reimbursed, but when people have lost the ability to swallow due to dementia, feeding tubes are devastating to their quality of life. Side effects include delirium, bedsores, agitation, and swelling. Many patients must be drugged or tied down to prevent them from pulling the tubes out. Their use in patients with end stage dementia, especially in those who have someone to speak for them, is declining.

Frailty: Physical fragility shown by slowing down, needing help from others, and losing resilience. Those with "mild frailty" need help with shopping and bill paying. Those with "moderate frailty" also need help with cooking meals, climbing stairs, and keeping house. Those with severe frailty are completely dependent on others, but in seemingly stable health. Those with "advanced frailty," described as "very severely frail," could not recover from even a minor illness and are likely to die within six months.

Frequent flyer: Crude hospital slang for a frail older person who repeatedly comes to the emergency room. Also called a crock, a crumble, or a GOMER (Get Out of My Emergency Room.)

Geriatrician: A specialist in the health problems of older people. A valuable, poorly paid, and endangered species.

Goals of care: How medicine might help you accomplish what matters most to you when cure is not a realistic hope. If a doctor wants to discuss "goals of care," it usually means that he or she thinks it's time to shift from cure-oriented, sometimes grueling treatments to relieving your suffering, finding out how you would define a good quality of life now, and preparing for the best possible death.

High-value care: A philosophy of medical reform, judging performance not by the number of tests or procedures performed, but by whether or not the patient actually gets healthier. Similar in approach to patient-centered care or person-centered care, but more concerned with cost.

Hospice: Taken from the French word for a medieval inn sheltering travelers and religious pilgrims, the word now has three interrelated English meanings. The original definition is a freestanding residence for the care of dying people. The second is the philosophy and practice of attending to the physical, emotional, medical, and spiritual needs of people approaching the end of life. The third, in the United States, is an insurance benefit providing a package of medical services to people in the last six months of life. Hospice nurses, social workers, doctors, and chaplains visit patients in private homes, nursing homes, hospitals, or freestanding residential hospices. Their focus is on relieving suffering, supporting caregivers, controlling pain, and providing spiritual, emotional, and physical comfort. To be eligible for the Medicare hospice benefit, people must agree to stop all curative treatments.

Some private insurance covers a full year "on hospice" and allows parallel use of some curative treatments.

Hospital delirium: Confusion, memory loss, and hallucinations that result from the stress of illness or a hospital stay. It was once thought to be a temporary state, but those who suffer it are at increased risk of developing dementia, of dying within a year, and of permanently losing mental function.

IADLs: Instrumental activities of daily living. See **ADLs**.

ICD: An implanted cardiac device. See **pacemaker** or **defibrillator**.

"I don't have a crystal ball": A phrase used by doctors to express uncertainty and discomfort when asked where things are heading, or how much time is left. Ask for a sketch of the typical course of your illness, and whether you have "days, weeks, months, or years." Further precision is rarely accurate.

Incurable: A word doctors now rarely use, preferring "chronic," "progressive," or "terminal."

Law of double effect: A moral principle articulated by the medieval Catholic theologian St. Thomas Aquinas, declaring that actions should be judged by their primary purpose, even if they also unintentionally cause a lesser harm. This "law" is widely used to justify giving morphine to the dying to relieve pain, even if, by depressing breathing, it may slightly hasten death.

Medical aid in dying (MIA): Proponents' phrase for legalizing the right of terminally ill people to obtain lethal prescriptions to time their deaths. Also called end-of-life options, the right to die, death with dignity, and physician-assisted dying.

Medical Power of Attorney: See **POA** or **Proxy**.

Metastases or Mets: Cancers that have spread to new places in the body, a sign the disease has progressed to stage four, is incurable, and will eventually be fatal.

MOLST (Medical Orders for Life-Sustaining Treatment): Signed by a doctor and more likely to be honored than an **advance directive**, a MOLST lists detailed treatments to be allowed or avoided. An invaluable document for anyone in the last years of life, or with an incurable illness. See also **POLST**.

Moral distress: The emotional and spiritual pain of medical staff forced, by hospital protocols or by patients' families, to do things to patients that cause suffering and violate the clinician's moral values. Often used to describe the anguish of nurses attending patients who are slowly and painfully dying in an ICU.

Multiple co-morbidities: Coexisting incurable, worsening illnesses, such as diabetes plus heart disease plus emphysema. Surgical risks rise exponentially, and the long-term outlook is poor.

Multiple organ systems failure: Organs vital to sustaining life (such as the liver, kidneys, lungs, and brain) are shutting down. Sometimes a medical euphemism for "dying," and often a precursor to it.

Nosocomial (condition): A health problem (including death or disability) caused by hospital treatment, including medication mixups, avoidable "complications" after surgery, hospital-acquired infections, and hospital delirium. Synonym: iatrogenic.

Overdiagnosis: Calling a physical condition a "disease" and treating it, even if it doesn't make you feel ill and will never do so, because of a non-normal or elevated result on a health **screening**, such as a PSA, blood, or thyroid test. Improved imaging has lowered the "thresholds of normality" for many conditions. Overdiagnosis wastes money and time, causes unnecessary worry, and frequently leads to **overtreatment**.

Overtreatment: Tests, drugs, and treatments that do more harm than good, because the "cure" exposes the patients to worse risks than the "disease" ever would. Treatment to satisfy a need or goal of someone other than the patient. "Treating the test" rather than the person.

Pacemaker: An implanted device delivering regular, painless, tiny electrical pulses to the heart, to correct a slow pulse. They can improve quality of life by lessening fatigue and fainting. But they may also prolong the dying process and are unnecessary in the absence of symptoms. (See, "treating the test.") If you are contemplating a pacemaker, it is important to discuss, with your doctor or nurse, an "exit plan" for painless nonsurgical deactivation when the device no longer serves your purposes. According to ethical statements issued by the major cardiology associations, deactivating a pacemaker is neither assisted suicide nor euthanasia. The decision is the patient's to make.

Palliative care: Medical care focused on relieving suffering and maintaining function, not on curing. Unlike hospice, it is appropriate at early stages of a serious or incurable illness, and can provide you with extra support, in parallel with cure-oriented treatments. It can help you maintain function, live a life worth living, and make empowered, informed decisions about your future medical care. In some health systems, palliative care is called supportive care, pain management, serious illness management, pre-hospice, or symptom management. Palliative care is not restricted to people within six months of dying who give up curative treatments. But it is often confused with hospice, because in some medical systems "palliative care" unfortunately means little more than having a doctor hold a last-minute conversation about disconnecting life support.

Palliative chemotherapy and palliative radiation: These are treatments intended to manage symptoms but not to cure. Palliative radiation effectively reduces or eliminates pain from cancers that have spread to the bone. So-called palliative chemotherapy sometimes negatively affects quality of life.

Patient representative: Hospital staff member charged with acting as a liaison and representing your concerns. If you have questions, complaints, or problems during a hospital stay, ask to see a patient representative, or the **charge nurse**.

Patient-centered care or person-centered care: Another medical reform movement, intended to put the needs of the patient, rather than the convenience of doctors, nurses, and health systems, at the center of medical treatment and decision-making.

Physician's order: A plan for treatment signed by a doctor and usually followed by other doctors and nurses. A physician's order or referral is required for a **do-not-resuscitate order** or a **POLST**, and to qualify for physical therapy, home health aides, and many other services reimbursed by Medicare or Medicaid.

POA: Power of attorney. Shorthand for medical power of attorney, or durable power of attorney for health care, this is the person you have designated to be your medical advocate. Also called your **Proxy**, Health Care Agent, or **Surrogate**.

POLST (Physician Orders for Life-Sustaining Treatment): A detailed doctor's order of medical treatments to be allowed or prohibited. Also known as **MOLST**. Most useful for people with terminal illnesses or in frail health, and more widely respected than **advance directives**.

Post-Operative Cognitive Decline (POCD): A loss of mental function, sometimes temporary and sometime permanent, after surgery. The risk of POCD rises with age, especially for those with existing cognitive impairments, and after open-heart surgery, general anesthesia, and hip replacement.

Primary care doctor: A generalist, usually an internist, who provides continuing care, hopefully knows the patient well, and writes referrals for services such as physical or occupational therapy.

Prognosis: A forecast of the usual course of your illness. In practice, prognosis often means bad news, and is often paired with words like "dire" or "poor."

Progressive: Medicalese for "it gets worse with time." Usually used at early stages of an incurable illness.

Proxy: Your medical advocate or health care agent, also known as your "surrogate," POA, or "medical power of attorney." This is the person you appoint to speak for you if you can't make medical decisions on your own. He or she should know your values and is legally charged with carrying out your previously expressed wishes. If your wishes are unknown, your proxy is required to decide in light of what he or she considers your best interests. If you have no proxy, doctors will usually recognize a close family member, or decide on the basis of whatever they consider your best interests. People without a proxy are more likely to be given treatments to sustain life rather than to allow a natural death.

Quality of life: Medical shorthand for "a life worth living," a highly individual matter. An acceptable quality of life to one person may be unacceptable to another. In medicine, quality of life traditionally includes health, well-being, life satisfaction, freedom from pain and suffering, and the ability to pursue enjoyed activities and to create meaning and connect with others. Any proposed treatment should be weighed in light of its effect on your quality of life—as you define it. If you or someone you love is receiving treatment that is increasing suffering with little hope of benefit, tell the medical team "I am concerned about quality of life."

Response rate: The percentage of people who have a positive result from a treatment. If you are told that a treatment has a good "response rate," ask what proportion of those treated have benefited, and whether that benefit translates into "clinical effectiveness" (direct improvement in your well-being or length of life) rather than "surrogate effectiveness" (shrinkage of your tumor or improvement on another test).

Risk management: A hospital legal division devoted to avoiding lawsuits. To get a hospital administration's attention, ask to speak with this department.

Screenings: The search for health problems in the absence of symptoms. Often leads to **overdiagnosis** and **overtreatment**. A full list of screenings not recommended is on the "Choosing Wisely" website of the American Board of Internal Medicine. (A diagnostic test, in contrast, is performed to find out the cause of a symptom and is more likely to be medically and practically useful.)

Sepsis: A catastrophic, whole-body, life-threatening, inflammatory response to infection. A common cause of ICU death.

Shared, collaborative, and informed medical decision-making: An attempt to shift the balance of power between patients and doctors by giving patients more information and agency, encouraging them to make their medical decisions in light of their preferences, values, and expectations. Assumes that there is no one right answer, and that several equally valid choices can be made, depending on the patient's priorities, needs, and risk tolerance. At its best, informed decision-making is a collaborative process, with doctors making clear recommendations based on their specialized knowledge and their understanding of the individual patient. At its worst, it devolves into a cafeteria-style conversation, with doctors simply offering a menu, as though surgery were the equivalent of selling a new car to an informed consumer. Also called medical decision-coaching.

Slow Medicine: A medical philosophy, movement, and practice that advocates giving doctors the time to make a careful diagnosis, to consider the needs and vulnerabilities of the whole patient, and to form a healing relationship. A reaction against "fast medicine," the hasty overprescribing of tests and treatments. One of its slogans is "To do more is not necessarily to do better." Started in Italy, it is now an international movement for medical reform.

SNF: A "sniff" is a skilled nursing facility, or Medicare-approved nursing home.

Stage four cancer: Cancer that has spread, or metastasized. It is almost never curable, though it sometimes can be slowed or managed.

Surrogate: See **Proxy**.

Surrogate effectiveness: Improvement in scores on a diagnostic test, under the assumption that these "surrogate markers" will translate into improved health, function, or length of life. They often don't.

Syncope: Fainting.

Terminal: Fatal and incurable. Your doctor would not be surprised if you died within six months.

Terminal, Total or Palliative sedation: keeping a dying patient unconscious until death comes, to soothe intractable agitation or pain. A sedative is administered via infusion or a specialized catheter.

Vertigo: Dizziness.

VSED (voluntary stopping of eating and drinking): Refusing food and water, or fasting, until death. It is legally permitted, in every state, but only for people who still have mental capacity.

"We have more arrows in our quiver": A phrase used by doctors meaning that the first or second treatments have stopped working, but he or she is willing to keep trying new drugs. Often used about stage four cancer and other diseases that can be slowed but not stopped. A good time to ask for a consultation with a palliative care doctor.

"Withdrawing care": An insensitive phrase used by doctors to mean releasing the patient from a painful, death-prolonging technology, such as a ventilator. In reality, doctors continue to *care* for such patients, but shift goals to "comfort care."

Worsening: A plain word many doctors avoid, preferring the more obfuscating **progressive**.

Resources

Recommended Reading:
"AGS 2018 Updated Beers Criteria® for Potentially Inappropriate Medication Use in Older Adults." *Journal of the American Geriatrics Society* (JAGS).

Megory Anderson. *Sacred Dying: Creating Rituals for Embracing the End of Life* New York: Da Capo Press; Rev and Expanded edition, 2003 and *Sacred Dying Journal* (Brewster, MA: Paraclete Press, 2018). Beautiful guides to creating simple rites of passage and spiritually preparing for a good end of life.

Elizabeth Bailey. *The Patient's Checklist: 10 Simple Hospital Checklists to Keep You Safe, Sane & Organized.* New York: Sterling Publishing, 2012. If a frail person must enter the hospital, this is the book to use.

Jari Holland Buck. *Hospital Stay Handbook: A Guide to Becoming a Patient Advocate for Your Loved Ones.* Woodbury, MN: Llewellyn Publications, 2007.

Ira Byock, MD. *Dying Well: Peace and Possibilities at the End of Life.* New York: Riverhead Books, 1998.

Roz Chast. *Can't We Talk About Something More Pleasant? A Memoir.* New York: Bloomsbury USA; Reprint edition 2016. Graphic memoir of caring for aging parents, with honesty and humor.

Hank Dunn. *Hard Choices for Loving People: Feeding Tubes, Palliative Care, Comfort Measures, and the Patient with a Serious Illness,* 6th edition. Naples, FL: Quality of Life Publishing Co., 2016. *The* guide to difficult medical decisions.

Atul Gawande. *Being Mortal: Medicine and What Matters in the End.* New York: Picador, 2017.

Joan Halifax. *Being with Dying: Cultivating Compassion and Fearlessness in the Presence of Death.* Boston: Shambhala; Reprint edition 2009.

K. Gabriel Heiser. *How to Protect Your Family's Assets from Devastating Nursing Home Costs: Medicaid Secrets.* Laredo, TX: Phylius Press, 2017.

Hospice Foundation of America. *The Dying Process: A Guide for Caregivers.* Free pamphlet.

Derek Humphries. *Final Exit: The Practicalities of Self-Deliverance and Assisted Suicide for the Dying.* New York: Delta Trade Paperback, 2010.

Barbara Karnes, RN. *Gone from My Sight: The Dying Experience.* Vancouver, WA: Barbara Karnes Publishing. A pamphlet describing the signs of approaching death.

David Kessler. *The Needs of the Dying: A Guide for Bringing Hope, Comfort and Love to Life's Final Chapter.* New York: Harper Perennial, 2007.

Judith Redwing Keyssar. *Last Acts of Kindness: Lessons for the Living from the Bedsides of the Dying.* Transformations-in-Care, 2010.

Dennis McCullough. *My Mother, Your Mother: Embracing "Slow Medicine," The Compassionate Approach to Caring for Your Aging Loved Ones.* New York: Harper Perennial, 2009.

Merck Manual of Geriatrics. West Point, PA: Merck (2000). Edited by Robert Berkow and Mark H. Beers. Detailed, helpful, and readable by educated laypeople.

Merck Manual of Health & Aging: The Comprehensive Guide to the changes and challenges of aging—for older adults and those who care for and about them. New York: Ballantine Books, 2005. Edited by Mark H. Beers. The layperson's version of the *Merck Manual of Geriatrics,* with similar information and a simpler reading level. Very useful.

Emmett Miller, MD. *Healing Journey.* A guided imagery audio for healing and relaxation. CD or MP3 from Drmiller.com; as an e-book at audiobooks.com.

Virginia Morris. *How to Care for Aging Parents: A One-Stop Resource for All Your Medical, Financial, Housing and Emotional Issues.* New York: Workman Publishing Company, 3rd edition, 2014. This, to my mind, is the best of the encyclopedic guides.

Frank Osasteski. *The Five Invitations.* New York: Flatiron Press, 2017. Spiritual guidance from the cofounder of San Francisco Zen hospice.

Physician's Desk Reference. Whippany, NJ: PDR Network 2016. Encyclopedia of medications, their purposes, and their side effects.

Phyllis Shacter. *Choosing to Die: A Personal Story. Elective Death by Voluntarily Stopping Eating and Drinking (VSED) in the Face of Degenerative Disease.* CreateSpace Independent Publishing Platform, 2017.

Elaine St. James. *Simplify Your Life: 100 Ways to Slow Down and Enjoy the Things That Really Matter* (New York: Hyperion, 2000). Not specifically for older people, but full of suggestions that prove helpful in coping with aging. See also, Elaine St. James,

Simplify Your Work Life (New York: Hyperion, 2001) and *Inner Simplicity* (New York: Hyperion, 1995).

Victoria Sweet. *God's Hotel* (New York: Riverhead Books, 2018) and *Slow Medicine* (New York: Riverhead Books, 2017). Brilliant, beautifully written first-person expositions of the philosophy of Slow Medicine, through the eyes of a talented physician-writer.

Bart Windrum. *The Promised Landing: A Gateway to Peaceful Dying.* Boulder, CO: Axiom Action, 2018. Brilliant analysis of the pathways of modern dying.

Films:

Alive Inside: A Story of Music and Memory. Directed by Michael Rossato-Bennett. Park City: Projector Media, 2014. About the healing power of music for people with dementia. Available on Amazon Video, Google Play, iTunes, Netflix, and YouTube.

Departures. Directed by Yojiro Takita. Montreal: Amuse Soft Entertainment, 2008. Beautiful Japanese movie about honoring the dead, told through the eyes of a young Buddhist cellist who takes a job as an undertaker. Available on Amazon Video, Google Play, iTunes, and YouTube.

Extremis. Directed by Dan Krauss. New York: f/8 Filmworks, 2016. Short documentary about life-and-death decisions in an intensive care unit at an Oakland, California, safety-net hospital. Featuring Dr. Jessica Nutik Zitter, a palliative care and ICU physician. Available on Netflix and YouTube.

Wit. Directed by Mike Nichols. Berlin: Avenue Pictures Productions, 2001. An English literature professor, dying alone in a hospital of metastatic ovarian cancer, seeks solace in John Donne while wrestling with institutional silence. Available on Amazon Video, HBO, and YouTube.

Further Sources of Reliable, Unbiased Medical Information:
American Cancer Society: at cancer.org. Unlike many promotional "disease foundations" funded by pharmaceutical companies, the ACS presents straightforward information and truly represents cancer patients.

Center for Science in the Public Interest: Excellent guides to medications.

Choosing Wisely: The American Board of Internal Medicine (ABIM) lists medical screenings and treatments that specialists say can be futile, risky, unnecessary, or otherwise do more harm than good. http://www.choosingwisely.org.

Cochrane Library: Nonbiased online reviews that compile evidence-based research on the effectiveness of many drugs and medical treatments, produced by a cooperative consortium of researchers. cochranelibrary.com.

Palliative Care of Wisconsin. Check their "Fast Facts" to learn what it is like to die from a specific disease, and how to manage its symptoms. mypcnow.org.

Drugs.com: Enter all your prescriptions and get a free, personalized report of possible interactions. https://www.drugs.com.

ePrognosis: Calculate the odds of how much time you have left: http://eprognosis.ucsf.edu/calculators.

Mayo Clinic: Reliable summaries of diseases and standard treatments. It's my first "go-to." http://www.mayoclinic.org.

MedShadow: Patients and health care providers discuss side effects of prescription medications. https://medshadow.org.

Number Needed to Treat (NNT): Run by physicians, NNT displays the proportion of people who will theoretically benefit from a drug or treatment, and the proportion who will suffer a side effect. It runs no advertisements and takes no pharmaceutical industry money. http://www.thennt.com.

UpToDate.com: Another well-vetted site for weighing the risks and benefits of treatments and medications. Built for physicians but readable by laypeople, it is backed by nonpartisan, noncommercial research. https://www.uptodate.com/home.

Worst Pills Best Pills: Neutral guidance on medication risks. http://www.worstpills.org.

Community Groups:

211: This line can be dialed direct in many areas for referrals to practical support services such as Meals on Wheels.

Alcoholics Anonymous: https://www.aa.org. See local listings in the White Pages for this free mutual support group, and others like it, including Food Addicts in Recovery Anonymous, Smokers Anonymous, and Overeaters Anonymous.

Area Agency on Aging: This local county agency is the first stop to search for services.

Centers for Medicare and Medicaid Services (CMS): Good website guide to Medicare basics at Medicare.gov.

Compassion and Choices: A group that promotes physician-assisted "right to die" legislation. It also has an excellent advice line for people resisting various forms of unwanted medical care.

Family Caregiver Alliance (Caregiver.org.): Political advocacy and referral to resources.

Get Palliative Care.org: Source for finding a palliative care practitioner by zip code. https://getpalliativecare.org.

Hospice Compare: Find local hospices, and compare their consumer satisfaction ratings at https://www.medicare.gov/hospice compare.

Hospice Foundation of America: Information and referrals to local hospices.

Judy MacDonald Johnston's "Prepare for a Good End of Life" TED Talk and website: Her excellent, reassuring checklist for preparing for a good end of life, is available at goodendoflife.com.

Lown Institute: This reformist medical group is concerned with overtreatment, overcharging, and other forms of non-patient-centered medicine.

Medicare Rights Center: Advocacy group with great website offering plain English explanations of Medicare coverage and benefits. 800-333-4114. Medicareinteractive.org.

Mindfulness Based Stress Reduction (MBSR): meditation courses are offered at many hospitals and useful in reducing chronic pain.

Sharethecare.org: Terrific guide to arranging practical volunteer support for chronically and terminally ill people. https://sharethe care.org.

Slow Medicine on Facebook: Closed, confidential discussion group, founded by Katy Butler, for family caregivers, gravely ill people, and professionals ranging from home health aides to hospice palliative care doctors and nurses. https://www.facebook.com.

State Health Insurance Assistance Program (SHIP): Funded by federal agencies and not affiliated with the insurance industry, this free counseling service can help you pick a Medicare insurance plan and access its benefits. A state-by-state list of SHIP programs is at the Seniors Resource Guide website: (seniors resourceguide.com/National/SHIP).

The Villages Movement: A mutual help network for older people who want to age in place. Villagetovillage.org.

Blogs and Online Magazines:

GeriPal blog: Geriatrics and palliative care blog for medical professionals; also useful to laypeople. http://www.geripal.org.

KevinMD (on MedPage Today): Honest essays about doctors' dilemmas, widely read and shared by medical professionals. http://www.kevinmd.com/blog.

NextAvenue.org: Excellent PBS online magazine covering health and aging.

Verywell.com: Excellent information on managing chronic illnesses.

Further Resources by Chapter:

CHAPTER 1: *Resilience*

Dan Buettner, *The Blue Zones Solution: Eating and Living Like the World's Healthiest People,* National Geographic reprint edition 2017.

Chris Crowley and Henry S. Lodge, MD, *Younger Next Year: Live Strong Fit and Sexy Until You're 80 and Beyond.* Workman, 2007.

Jane Fonda, YouTube exercise videos for older people. https://www.youtube.com/user/janefondatv.

Dr. Dean Ornish, *Dr. Dean Ornish's Program for Reversing Heart Disease: The Only System Scientifically Proven to Reverse Heart Disease Without Drugs or Surgery,* Ivy Books, 1995.

Michael Pollan, *Food Rules: An Eater's Manual,* Penguin Books, 2009.

Royal Canadian Air Force Exercise Plans for Physical Fitness, Echo Point Books & Media, reprint edition 2016. A favorite of actress Helen Mirren, these aerobic and strength-training exercises are doable anywhere without special equipment or expertise, and take no more than twenty minutes per day.

CHAPTER 2: *Slowing Down*

Drugs containing brain-threatening anticholinergics

- Sleep remedies: Benadryl, Sominex, Excedrin PM, Advil PM, Aleve PM, Nytol, Simply Sleep, Tylenol PM, and anything else containing diphenhydramine.
- Allergy remedies: Actifed, Chlor-Trimeton, Codeprex, Advil Allergy and Congestion Relief, and others containing chlorpheniramine Antihistamines (Loratadine, CopheneB, Bromax) containing brompheniramine.
- Muscle relaxants containing cyclobenzaprines (Amrix, Fexmid, Flexeril).
- Bladder control drugs containing oxybutynin (Ditropan, Oxytrol).
- Antispasmodics for irritable bowel: (Belladonna, Donnatal, Librax, Bentyl).

Other prescription drugs dangerous to the elderly

- Old-school tricyclic antidepressants (Elavil, doxepin, Sinequan). Alternatives are SSRIs like Prozac if tolerated (though they also pose fall risks), bupropion (Wellbutrin), or Buspar (buspirone).

- Benzodiazepines like Librium, Ativan, and Xanax, prescribed for anxiety, can worsen delirium and contribute to unsteady gait, fainting, falls, accidents, and fractures. Taper off slowly under medical supervision. (These drugs, however, can be helpful when on hospice.)
- Sleep drugs: Ambien, barbiturates, chloral hydrate, Lunesta, Sonata, Zaleplon, and Zolpidem all increase risks of cognitive impairment, delirium, unsteady gait, falls, fainting, and car accidents.

All are on the "Beers List" of drugs potentially harmful to the elderly, regularly updated by the American Geriatrics Society, and summarized well at Pharmacist's Letter/Prescriber's Letter (pharmacistsletter.com).

The Conversation Project (theconversationproject.com) has downloadable "Starter Kits" to help you open up discussions of end-of-life medical choices with family and friends. I especially recommend their guide for exploring issues involving dementia. https://theconversationproject.org/starter-kits/.

CHAPTER 3: *Adaptation*

The following HMOs and Medicare Advantage plans provide well-coordinated medical care and are highly rated:

- CareMore Health Systems throughout California
- Geisinger Health Systems in Pennsylvania and New Jersey
- Kaiser Permanente in many states
- Optum Healthcare and ProHealth in Florida
- Sharp Rees-Stealy in San Diego, California
- Bon Secours in Richmond, Virginia
- Meridian Health in Hackensack, New Jersey
- Intermountain Healthcare in Utah and Idaho
- OSF Medical Group in Morton, Illinois
- University of Pittsburgh Medical Center

- University of Alabama at Birmingham, Center for Palliative and Supportive Care

The **National Library Service** provides free braille and talking books and magazines, by mail and via downloads, for people with low vision, blindness, or physical disability that prevents them from reading or holding the printed page. https://www.loc.gov/nls.

This Caring Home offers adaptive home appliances, including stoves that turn off automatically to reduce the risk of fire. http://www.thiscaringhome.org.

Marinvillages.org and **techenhancedlife.com** provide fall-proofing checklists to help older adults remain safely at home. http://marinvillages.org and https://www.techenhancedlife.com.

The Village to Village movement will help you find a network of mutual support in your area, or help you start your own. www.vtvnetwork.org.

K. Gabriel Heiser's *How to Protect Your Family's Assets from Devastating Nursing Home Costs: Medicaid Secrets* is an excellent guide to preparing financially for Medicaid.

CHAPTER 4: *Awareness of Mortality*
Ira Byock, MD. *The Four Things That Matter Most: A Book About Living,* 10th anniversary edition. New York: Atria Books, 2014.

CHAPTER 5: *House of Cards*
The following organizations are national leaders in home-based medical care:

- Aspire Healthcare, an add-on offered by health plans in many states
- Doctors on Call, Brooklyn, New York
- House Call Providers, Portland, Oregon

- Boston Medical Center's House Call program, Boston, Massachusetts
- Christiana Health Services, Wilmington, Delaware
- Cleveland Clinic Home Care Services, Independence, Ohio
- Doctors Making House calls, Durham, North Carolina
- Med Star Washington Hospital Center, Washington, D.C.
- National House Call Practitioners Group, Austin, Texas
- North Shore Long Island Jewish Health Care's Physician House calls Program, Westbury, New York
- UCSF Medical Center Geriatrics Department, San Francisco, California
- University of Pennsylvania Health System House Call Program
- Veterans Administration's Home Based Primary Care program (HBPC)
- Virginia Commonwealth University programs in Pennsylvania, Virginia, and Washington, D.C.
- Visiting Physicians Associations in Dallas, Texas; Flint and Lansing, Michigan; Jacksonville, Florida; and Milwaukee, Wisconsin

CHAPTER 6: *Preparing for a Good Death*

Ira Byock, *Dying Well: Peace and Possibilities at the End of Life* (New York: Riverhead Books, 1998).

Cappy Caposella and Sheila Warnock, *Share the Care: How to Organize a Group to Care for Someone Who Is Seriously Ill* (New York: Fireside, 2004), and the website, Sharethecare.org.

Margareta Magnusson, *The Gentle Art of Swedish Death Cleaning: How to Free Yourself and Your Family from a Lifetime of Clutter* (New York: Scribner, 2018).

Notes

xi   *"I worried"*: From *Swan*, Beacon Press © 2012, Mary Oliver and Beacon Press. Reprinted by permission.

INTRODUCTION: *The Lost Art of Dying*

1 *favorite daughter Mary*: Family history drawn from the diaries of Philippa Norman Butler and her daughter-in-law, Marie Watts Butler, and from *Karoo Morning* by Guy Butler (David Philip Publishers, South Africa, 1982).

2 *upper reaches*: The exceptions are violence, suicide, accidents, and drug overdoses, the major causes of death in the U.S. prior to the age of forty-five.

3 *"habits of the heart"*: This phrase, coined by Alexis de Tocqueville to describe the customs and ceremonies of daily life, was popularized by sociologist Robert Bellah in *Habits of the Heart: Individualism and Commitment in American Life* (University of California Press, 1985, 2007).

3 *sixty-five editions*: Philip Meggs, et al. *Megg's History of Graphic Design* (Wiley and Sons, 2016), Figs. 7–14.

3 *Ars Moriendi*: My summary is drawn from William Rylands and George, Bullen, eds. *The Ars Moriendi, Editio Princeps, Circa 1450, A Reproduction of the Copy in the British Museum* (Wyman and Sons, London, 1881); William Caxon and Heinrich Seuse, *The Book of the Craft of Dying and Other Early English Tracts Concerning Death*, edited by Frances Comper (Longmans, Green, London, 1917); and Nancy Lee Beaty, *The Craft of Dying: The Literary Tradition of the Ars Moriendi in England* (Yale University Press, 1970).

5 *three-quarters of Americans*: Liz Hamel et al, "Views and Experiences with End of Life Care in the US," *Henry J. Kaiser Family Foundation*, in partnership with *The Economist*, April 27, 2017.

5 *fewer than a third*: Centers for Disease Control, WONDER database, accessed January 28, 2016. http://wonder.cdc.gov.

5 *die in an ICU*: Joan M. Teno, et al., "Change in End-of-Life Care for Medicare Beneficiaries," *JAMA* 309, No. 5 (February 6, 2013). Susan W. Tolle and Joan M. Teno, et al., "Lessons from Oregon in Embracing Complexity in End-of-Life Care," *N Engl J M* 376, no. 11. (March 16 2017), Fig. 1., p. 1079.

5 *"torture"*: See Jessica Nutik Zitter, MD, *Extreme Measures: Finding a Better Path to the End of Life* (Penguin Random House, 2017).

5 *is intensifying*: Last-minute hospice enrollment is increasing, but so is the proportion of people who spend time in an ICU in their final month.

6 *assembly line*: The metaphor of the "end-of-life conveyor belt" was formulated by Jessica Nutik Zitter, MD, in *Extreme Measures* (Avery, 2017). I first came across the metaphor of hospitals as "body repair shops" in Bart Windrum's *Notes from the Waiting Room: Managing a Loved One's End-of-Life Hospitalization* (Axiom Action, 2008). A similar metaphor is used by Victoria Sweet, MD, in *Slow Medicine: The Way to Healing* (Riverhead Books, 2017).

7 *A 2017 poll*: Liz Hamel et al, "Views and Experiences with End of Life Care in the US," *Henry J. Kaiser Family Foundation*, in partnership with *The Economist*, April 27, 2017.

9 *"a gentle, mild and sweet"*: Schulz, Zacharias Philipp/Alberti, Michael, *De euthanasia medica, Vom leichten Todt*, diss., U. of Halle 1735, p.10. CF Michael Stolberg, *A History of Palliative Care 1500–1970: Concepts, Practices, and Ethical Challenges* (Springer, 2017). p.33.

CHAPTER 1: *Resilience*

12 "The River Grows Wider": From Bertrand Russell, *Portraits from Memory and Other Essays* (Allen and Unwin, 1951).

15 *cardiac rehabilitation*: People who participate suffer fewer deaths from heart disease, are less likely to be hospitalized, and report better psychological health and quality of life. See Hasnain M. Dalal, Patrick Doherty, and Rod S. Taylor. "Cardiac Rehabilitation," *BMJ (Clinical Research Ed.)* 351 (2015):500; and Dean Ornish, et al., "Intensive Lifestyle Changes for Reversal of Coronary Heart Disease," *JAMA* 280, no. 23 (1998):2001–2007.

15 *halved Doug's risk*: A study of over 30,000 heart patients found that those who changed their diet, exercised more, and didn't smoke were half as likely to die within five years of a first episode, or suffer another heart attack than were sedentary smokers who ate a lot of meat., J. Booth, et al., "Effect of Sustaining Lifestyle Modifications," *Am J Cardiol* 113 no. 12 (June 2014):1933–1940.

16 *by a fall*: People over seventy who regularly practice t'ai chi are half as likely to fall as those who don't, and half as likely to be injured if they do fall.

16 *major threats*: Neil Mehta, and Mikko Myrskyla, "The Population Health Benefits of a Healthy Lifestyle: Life Expectancy Increased and Onset of Disability Delayed," *Health Affairs* 36, no. 8 (2017).

16 *prolong your time in Resilience*: Mark Hamer, et al., "Taking up physical activity in later life and healthy ageing [sic]: the English longitudinal study of ageing," *British Journal of Sports Medicine*, 48, no. 3 (February 2014). People who started exercising after age fifty-five had a sevenfold reduction in their risk of becoming ill or infirm eight years later.

17 *spiritual and social strength*: Group support to change life habits is available at Diabetes Prevention classes, offered at more than two hundred Ys around the country and covered by Medicare because they are effective. Others find success in free twelve-step support groups like Alcoholics Anonymous, Smokers Anonymous, Overeaters Anonymous, and Food Addicts in Recovery Anonymous.

18 *break a sweat*: In a study at the University of Pittsburgh, sixty sedentary older adults walked together several times a week, briskly enough to break a sweat. After one year, their hippocampuses had grown by an average of 2 percent, more than reversing the brain cell loss recorded in normal aging. The hippocampuses of a comparison group who only did nonaerobic stretching and yoga shrank by the normal 2 percent. See Kirk I. Erickson, "Exercise training increases size of hippocampus and improves memory," *Proceedings of the National Academy of Sciences* 108, no. 7 (February 2011):3017–3022.

19 *"never going back"*: For those interested in lifestyle changes, I recommend three excellent books: *Younger Next Year, Food Rules,* and *Blue Zone Solutions,* a National Geographic–funded study of health habits common among cultures around the world where people tend to live long lives without developing dementia. All are listed in the resource section and favor a "non-Western diet" heavy in fruits and vegetables and low in processed foods. Researchers continue to confirm the magnitude of its positive effects on reducing cancer, heart disease, and other degenerative illnesses.

21 *"failed back surgery syndrome"*: See Cathryn Jakobson Ramin, *Crooked: Outwitting the Back Pain Industry and Getting on the Road to Recovery* (HarperCollins, 2017).

21 *with little vetting*: See Brent Ardaugh, et al., "The 510(k) Ancestry of a Metal-on-Metal Hip Implant," *N Engl J Med* 368 (January 2013):97–100.

22 *"postoperative cognitive impairment"*: Ingrid Rundshagen, "Postoperative Cognitive Dysfunction," *Dtsch Arztebl Int.* 111, no. 8 (February 2014):119–125.

26 *your legal and moral right*: Doctors cannot be forced to terminate a treatment if they consider it unethical to do so, but they are professionally obligated to refer you to a more sympathetic doctor.

28 *"Five Wishes"*: This document meets the legal requirements for advance directives in forty-two states and the District of Columbia. It is not legally approved in Alabama, Indiana, Kansas, New Hampshire, Ohio, Oregon, Texas, and Utah; people in these states should fill out the standard forms recognized there.

30 *handwriting a letter*: I suggest handwriting because it is easier to authenticate an entirely handwritten letter than a generic computer printout that is signed but not witnessed. In many states, handwritten (holographic) wills are legally binding even when not notarized or witnessed.

32 *"There is no way"*: This version of the "Five Remembrances" comes from the tradition of the Vietnamese Zen master Thich Nhat Hanh.

CHAPTER 2: *Slowing Down*

36 *the afternoon of life*: Carl Jung, *Collected Works,* vol. 8.

37 *following statements*: This list does not define a formal medical syndrome, but practical, commonsense signs of your current state of health, and the forms of medical care most likely to be helpful.

42 *"seldom 'fixed' by a drug"*: Dennis McCullough, *My Mother, Your Mother: Embracing "Slow Medicine," the Compassionate Approach to Caring for Your Aging Loved Ones* (Harper Perennial, 2009), p. 44.

42 *primary care physicians*: Comments section, Katy Butler, "Imagine a Medicare 'Part Q' for Quality at the End of Life," in The End, *New York Times,* December 9, 2015. https://opinionator.blogs.nytimes.com/2015/12/09/imagine-a-medicare-part-q-for-quality-at-the-end-of-life.

43 *All-under-one-roof HMOs*: In 2007, in the San Francisco Bay Area, where the Kaiser Permanente HMO dominates, people in Medicare Advantage plans spent one-third fewer days in the hospital than those in "original" fee-for-service Medicare.

45 *emergency room visits*: Daniel S. Budnitz, et al., "National Surveillance of Emergency Department Visits for Outpatient Adverse Drug Events," *JAMA* 295 (2006):1858–1866. doi: 10.1001/jama.296.15.1858.

45 *(and no other purpose)*: A thorough medication review will require at least a fifteen-minute appointment, and should not be combined with other health concerns.

46 *medication review*: Walgreens offers a medication review by a pharmacist to their prescription drug customers.

46 *Cholesterol lowering statins*: See the nonprofit, physician-run "Number Needed to Treat" website (www.thennt.com) which assesses drug treatments, runs no advertisements, and takes no pharmaceutical industry money.

46 *can cause kidney damage*: Mehul Dixit, et al., "Significant Acute Kidney Injury Due to Non-steroidal Anti inflammatory Drugs: Inpatient

Setting," *Pharmaceuticals* (Basel) 3, no. 4 (April 2010): 1279–1285. Published online April 26 2010.

47 Anticholinergics: American Geriatrics Society's "Beers List": Therapeutic Research Center, "Potentially Harmful Drugs in the Elderly: Beers List." Pharmacist's Letter/Prescriber's Letter June, 2012, updated 2015. Accessed February 18, 2016 at pharmacistsletter.com.

47 *develop dementia*: In 2015, researchers at the University of Washington School of Pharmacy studied the health records of three thousand people over sixty-five, all cognitively intact at the start of the study. Those who took anticholinergics daily for three years or more had a 54 percent greater risk of being diagnosed with dementia ten years later. Occasional use (five to ten times a year) did not increase risk. See Shelly L. Gray, et al., "Cumulative Use of Strong Anticholinergics and Incident Dementia: A Prospective Cohort Study," *JAMA Internal Medicine* 175, no. 3 (2015):401–407. dci: 10.1001/jamaintern med.2014.7663.

47 Benzodiazepines: Jennifer Glass, "Sedative Hypnotics in Older People with Insomnia: Meta-Analysis of Risks and Benefits," *BMJ* 31 (2005):1169. doi: 10.1136/bmj.38623.768588.47.

48 *relaxation or self-hypnosis audio*: I recommend Michael Sealey's free audios on YouTube, Emmett Miller, MD's, CD or MP3, "Healing Journey," and John Vosler, "Yoga Nidra."

49 *PSA (prostate cancer tests)*: See the Society for Post-Acute and Long-Term Care Medicine, "Don't Recommend Screening for Breast, Colorectal or Prostate Cancer If Life Expectancy Is Estimated to Be Less Than 10 Years," Choosing Wisely, last modified March 20, 2015, http://www.choosingwisely.org/clinician-lists.

49 *Colonoscopies*: The U.S. Preventive Services Task Force recommends no routine colon cancer screening for those older than seventy-five, and no screening at all for those over age eighty-five. Because polyps grow slowly, it's unlikely they'll develop into full-blown cancers before death arrives from another cause. See Paula Span, "Unnecessary Colon Screenings for Elderly Patients," New Old Age, *New York Times*, May 25, 2011, https://newoldage.blogs.nytimes.com/2011/05/25/un necessary-colon-screenings-for-elderly-patients.

50 *Antidepressants cannot cure*: The antidepressant Wellbutrin is sometimes better tolerated by older people.

50 *"hole in our home"*: I am grateful to Doug von Koss for permission to draw from his unpublished essay about this experience.

CHAPTER 3: *Adaptation*

55 *You may find this chapter*: The criteria for this chapter correspond roughly with mild to moderate frailty on the Clinical Frailty Scale.

58 *Marin Villages*: See Marin Villages website, marinvillages.org.

62 *prenuptial agreement*: Some couples faced with this dilemma get a legal "Medicaid divorce" to financially protect the healthy spouse.

64 *exercise class*: See "Jane Fonda: Fit and Strong Level 1," YouTube.

65 *Inside the house*: A thorough fall-proofing checklist is downloadable at www.Marinvillages.org and at www.techenhancedlife.org.

66 *occupational therapist*: Medicare requires a doctor's referral for occupational, speech, and physical therapy.

66 *Hearing aids*: Costco has good prices. A new generation of less expensive "Personal Amplification Devices," not regulated by the FDA, can do the job nearly as well.

69 *pay for some services*: Some religious and charitable groups, such as local Catholic Charities and Jewish Family and Children's Services agencies, offer services on a sliding scale, and you do not have to be of any particular religion to qualify. In your search for services, start with your county's Area Agency on Aging. Many areas also have a social services referral hotline: dial 211.

70 *Caregivers experience*: J. K. Monin, et al., "Spouses' Daily Feelings of Appreciation and Self-Reported Well Being," *Health Psychology* 36, no. 12 (December 2017).

72 *nursing homes*: Valery Hazanov, "What Working in a Nursing Home Taught Me about Life, Death, and America's Cultural Values," Vox (December 2, 2015). http://www.vox.com.

74 *t'ai chi*: This ancient "soft" martial art increases ankle flexibility and thigh and core body strength. Once only known in pockets of the country with many Asian residents, it is now offered in many senior centers and assisted living residences in the Midwest and elsewhere. A hands-on teacher is best, but the basics can be learned via the highly rated iTunes app for the iPhone, *T'ai Chi for Seniors*, by Discovery Publisher Limited.

CHAPTER 4: *Awareness of Mortality*

77 end stage: If doctors use the term "multiple organ systems failure," death is probably close, and the chapters "Preparing for a Good Death" and "Active Dying" will be more helpful.

82 *Ron Belcher, who was seventy-two*: "How patients make decisions about cancer care: The story of Ronnie Belcher," Stanford Ace Aging videotaped panel with Tim Belcher, V. J. Periakoyl, MD, and Charles Von Gunten, MD. https://aging.stanford.edu/2013/11/making-hard-decisions/part 1. Accessed Jan 2, 2018.

83 *fatal lung cancers*: H. A. Huskamp, et al., "Discussions with physicians about hospice among patients with metastatic lung cancer," *Arch Intern Med* 169, no. 10 (May 2009):954–962.

84 *mistaken impression*: J. C. Weeks, et al., "Patients' expectations about

effects of chemotherapy for advanced cancer," *N Engl J M* 367, no. 17 (October 2012):1616–25. doi: 10.1056/NEnglJM oa1204410.

84 *a clear understanding*: Jennifer W. Mack and Thomas J. Smith, "Reasons Why Physicians Do Not Have Discussions About Poor Prognosis, Why It Matters, and What Can Be Improved," *Journal of Clinical Oncology* 30, no. 22 (2012):2715–2717, doi: 10.1200/JCO.2012.42.4564; Thomas J. Smith, et al., "A Pilot Trial of Decision Aids to Give Truthful Prognostic and Treatment Information to Chemotherapy Patients with Advanced Cancer," *Journal of Supportive Oncology* 9, no. 2 (2011):79–86; and Andrew S. Epstein et al., "Discussions of Life Expectancy and Changes in Illness Understanding in Patients with Advanced Cancer," *Journal of Clinical Oncology* 34, no. 20 (2016):2398–2403. doi: 10.1200/JCO.2015.63.6696.

85 *overestimate their patients' survival times*: Nicholas A Christakis and Elizabeth B. Lamont, "Extent and determinants of error in doctors' prognoses in terminally ill patients: prospective cohort study," *BMJ* 320, no. 7233 (February 2000):469–473. On average, doctors overestimated survival length by a factor of 5.3.

86 *common trajectories*: All but the third trajectory, which is my own, were created by geriatrician Joanne Lynn and reprinted by Atul Gawande in *Being Mortal*. Joanne Lynn, "Living Long in Fragile Health: The New Demographics Shape End of Life Care," *Improving End of Life Care: Why Has It Been So Difficult? Hastings Center Special Report* 35, no. 6 (2005):S14–S18.

90 "*apalliating*" . . . "*by gentle remedies*": Giovanni da Vigo (1450–1525), *Chirurgerye* (first English translation, 1543.) CF Michael Stolberg, *A History of Palliative Care, 1500–1970: Concepts, Practices, and Ethical Challenges* (Springer, 2017) p. 21.

91 *American Heart Association*: Lynne T. Braun, et al., "Palliative Care and Cardiovascular Disease and Stroke: A Policy Statement from the American Heart Association/American Stroke Association." *Circulation* 134, no. 11 (September 2016):3198-e225, epublished August 8, 2018.

91 *American Society of Clinical Oncology*: Betty R. Ferrell, et al., "Integration of Palliative Care into Standard Oncology Care: American Society of Clinical Oncology Clinical Practice Guideline Update," 2016.

91 *often live longer*: Jennifer S. Temel, MD, et al., "Early Palliative Care for Patients with Metastatic Non-Small-Cell Lung Cancer." *N Engl J M* 363 (August 19, 2010):733–742. doi: 10.1056/ *N Engl J M* oa1000678.

92 *palliative care specialist*: Amy Berman. "A Nurse with Fatal Cancer Says End-of-Life Discussions Saved Her Life." *Washington Post*, June 1, 2016.

92 *a single carefully focused burst*: "Choosing Wisely" website of the American Board of Internal Medicine (ABIM).

92 *Jerry Romano*: "Preventing Deathbed Shocks: Jerry Romano's Story,"
Author interview with Soo-Ling Chang, 2016, and videotaped panel
discussion at Stanford University with Katy Butler, Dipanjan Banerjee,
MD, and V. J. Periakoyl, MD. Broadcast on YouTube and on "Ace Aging"
website, Stanford Medical School, Palo Alto, California, recorded September 2013. http://aging.stanford.edu/2013/11story-jerry-romano/
Accessed July 18 2016, no longer accessible. See also interview of Katy
Butler by V. J. Periakoyl, MD: https://aging.stanford.edu/2013/11
/knocking-heavens-door-conversation-katy-butler/.

94 *patient's survival time*: John Fauber and Elbert Chu, "The Slippery
Slope: Is a Surrogate Endpoint Evidence of Efficacy?" *Medpage Today*,
October 26, 2014, https://www.medpagetoday.com/special-reports
/slipperyslope/48244.

95 *the law of diminishing returns*: The American Society of Clinical Oncology (ASCO) does not recommend third and fourth lines of treatment for people with lung cancer and impaired health and function.
See ASCO NSCLC Decision Aid, ASCO 2009.

95 *fourth line produces*: Ashahina, et al. "Retrospective analysis of third-
line and fourth-line chemotherapy for advanced non-small-cell lung
cancer." *Clin Lung Cancer* 13, no. 1 (January 2012):39–43.

96 *"buy and bill"*: Blase Polite, MD, et al., "Reform of the Buy-and-Bill
System for Outpatient Chemotherapy Care Is Inevitable: Perspectives
from an Economist, a Realpolitik, and an Oncologist." *Am Soc Clin
Oncol Educ Book*, 2015.

98 *FDA never approves*: Jonathan Kimmelman, "Is Participation in Cancer Phase 1 Trials Really Therapeutic?" *J Clin Oncol* 35, no. 2 (January
2017):135–138. Published online September 30, 2016. doi: 10.1200
/JCO.2016.67.9902. Accessed January 18, 2018.

98 *5 percent . . . gained more time*: E. Horstmann, M. S. McCabe, et al.,
"Risks and benefits of phase I oncology trials, 1991 through 2002." *N
Engl J Med* 352, no. 9 (March 2005):895–904. See also, Anthony L.
Back, Wendy G. Anderson, et al., "Communication about cancer
near the end of life," *Cancer* 113, 7 Suppl (October 2008):1897–1910.
doi:10.1002/cncr.23653.

98 *"desperate patients"*: Jonathan Kimmelman, "Is Participation in Cancer
Phase 1 Trials Really Therapeutic?" *J Clin Oncol.* 35, no. 2 (January
2017):135–138. Published online September 30, 2016. doi: 10.1200
/JCO.2016.67.9902.

98 *"a scorched-earth operation"*: Siddhartha Mukherjee, "The Invasion
Equation," *The New Yorker* (September 17, 2017).

99 *frequently shortens life*: Holly G. Prigerson, et al., "Chemotherapy Use,
Performance Status, and Quality of Life at the End of Life," *JAMA Oncology* 1, no. 6 (2015):778–784. doi: 10.1001/jamaoncol.2015.2378.

99 *Cancerous tumors*: Siddhartha Mukherjee, "The Invasion Equation," *The New Yorker* (September 17, 2017).

99 *Marijuana for medical purposes*: Michael Stolberg, *A History of Palliative Care, 1500–1970: Concepts, Practices and Ethical Challenges* (Springer 2017), p. 102.

101 *Norma Jean Bauerschmidt*: Tim Bauerschmidt and Ramie Liddle, *Driving Miss Norma: One Family's Journey to Saying Yes to Living* (HarperOne, 2017).

CHAPTER 5: *House of Cards*

106 Although the Wind: Izumi Shikibu, "Although the wind . . . ," translated by Jane Hirshfield and Mariko Aratani, from *The Ink Dark Moon*, Vintage Classics, 1990. Reprinted by permission.

107 *of the following statements*: Statements two through eight on this list are formal criteria for a clinical diagnosis of "advanced frailty," characterized by weakness, slow movement, lack of stamina, weight loss, exhaustion, inactivity, and unsteady balance. Numerous studies have shown that frail people face greater risks from surgery and hospitalization, and so do people with several coexisting serious illnesses (multiple co-morbidities) such as diabetes plus heart trouble plus emphysema.

107 *"the dwindles"*: In the words of poet and longtime hospice volunteer Pam Heinrich MacPherson, "the dwindles" is a letting-go that "occurs in frail elders and moves slowly, only in one direction, i.e., toward life closure."

107 *more than twenty seconds*: This is known as the "Timed Up and Go" (TUG) test. If this test alone takes you more than twenty seconds, you meet the definition of frailty and are at high risk of falling or having complications after surgery.

107 *live in a nursing home*: If you answered "yes" to three or more of the statements two through eight, you officially meet the American Geriatrics Society's definition of frailty. You have a fifty-fifty chance of coming out worse, not better, from any hospital stay. The more "yes" statements you agree to, the greater your risks. See Daniel Hoefer, MD, "*If Only Someone Had Warned Us*," Coalition for Compassionate Care of California recorded webinar, accessed in 2015, http://coalitionccc.teachable.com/p/if-only-someone-had-warned-us.

108 *If Only Someone Had Warned Us*: Daniel Hoefer, MD, has heard this phrase from numerous families after disastrous hospitalizations.

109 *frail patients are more likely*: Martin A. Makary, et al., "Frailty as a Predictor of Surgical Outcomes in Older Patients," *Journal of the American College of Surgeons* 210, no. 6 (2010): 901–8. doi:10.1016/j.jamcollsurg.2010.01.028.

112　*age of eighty-one*: Linda Fried, et al., "Untangling the Concepts of Disability, Frailty and Comorbidity: Implications for Improved Targeting and Care," *Journals of Gerontology Series A: Biological Sciences and Medical Sciences* 59, no. 3 (2004):M255–M263. doi: 10.1093/gerona/59.3.M255.

113　*without house call services*: Many states require assisted living residents to get a medical assessment within twenty-four hours of any "change in health status," such as a fall. In places without onsite medical staff, this usually means a trip, warranted or not, to the emergency room. Meet with the home's medical or executive director and see if you can sign a waiver, make alternative medical arrangements such as a physician house call service, or get a "do not transport" medical order.

114　*keep patients out of the hospital*: Paula Span, "The Patient Wants to Leave. The Hospital Says, 'No Way.'" *New York Times,* July 7, 2017.

114　*emergency room only for things*: Symptoms of stroke include: facial drooping, a one-sided smile, slurred speech, or weakness, numbness or paralysis of one arm or leg. Clot-busting medications, administered early, can reduce permanent disability. Call 911, say "This is a stroke," and get to the front of the line.

116　*fifty thousand older people a year*: Carijn Lelieveld, et al., "Discharge Against Medical Advice Among Elderly Inpatients in the U.S.," *Journal of the American Geriatrics Society* 65, no. 9 (September 2017):2094–2099, epublished June 2017. doi:10.1111/jgs.14985.

117　*DASH*: Medicare and Medicaid reimbursed DASH on a fee-for-service basis, but didn't cover travel time or reimburse for communications with the patient's various doctors. Those significant costs were covered by charitable grants and the monthly fees paid by some patients.

118　*financially supported*: In 2016, in a pilot project called Independence at Home, Medicare provided additional funding to a selection of house call programs across the country with similarities to DASH. They are included in the resources section.

119　*POLST*: Sample copies and specific state regulations are available from POLST Paradigm at Polst.org. In 2018, about half of the states had POLST programs, and most others, with the exception of South Dakota and Washington, D.C., were developing them.

122　*benefit from palliative care*: Susan Mitchel, et al., "The Clinical Course of Advanced Dementia," *New Engl J Med* 361 (October 15, 2009):1595–1596.

123　*"Uncertainty is not"*: Zygmunt Bauman, *Alone Again: Ethics After Certainty* (Demos Press, 1994).

124　*draw out dying for weeks*: "End of Life Decisions," © 2016, Alzheimer's Association.

124　*For more detailed guidance*: See Hank Dunn, *Hard Choices for Loving People: Feeding Tubes, Palliative Care, Comfort Measures, and the Pa-*

tient with a Serious Illness, 6th edition (Naples: Quality of Life Publishing Co., 2016).

127 *letter I've written*: My letter was adapted from, and inspired by, an online version that I can no longer access.

129 *geriatrics specialists recommend*: A reminder: this loosening-up is relevant for frail people in the House of Cards, not necessarily for vigorous older people who still function well on their own.

129 *blood pressure*: Veronika van der Wardt, "Should Guidance for the Use of Antihypertensive Medication in Older People with Frailty Be Different?" *Age and Ageing* 44, no. 6 (2015):912–913. doi: https://doi .org/10.1093/ageing/afv147. See also Athenase Benetos, et al., "Polypharmacy in the Aging Patient: Management of Hypertension in Octogenarians." *JAMA* 314 (2015):170–180, doi: 10.1001/jama.2015.7517 and Michelle C. Odden, et al., "Rethinking the Association of High Blood Pressure with Mortality in Elderly Adults: The Impact of Frailty," *Archives of Internal Medicine* 172 (2012):1162–1168, doi: 10.1001 /archinternmed.2012.2555.

129 *Blood pressure medications*: Mary E. Tinetti, et al., "Antihypertensive Medications and Serious Fall Injuries in a Nationally Representative Sample of Older Adults." *JAMA Internal Medicine* 174, no. 4 (2014):588–595. doi: 10.1001/jamainternmed.2013.14764.

130 *Dietrich Mayer*: "Dietrich" and "Betty" are pseudonyms.

CHAPTER 6: *Preparing for a Good Death*

136 Awakened: Czeslaw Milosz, *Selected and Last Poems* (Ecco reprint edition, 2011). Reprinted by permission.

139 *palliative chemo*: Holly G. Prigerson, PhD, et al., "Chemotherapy Use, Performance Status, and Quality of Life at the End of Life." *JAMA Oncology* 1, no. 6 (2015):778–784. doi: 10.1001/jamaoncol.2015.2378.

143 *arrange an informational meeting*: You are most likely to die in the place where you are currently receiving your medical care. If hospice is not an option, explore a physician house call service, as discussed in Chapter 5, "House of Cards."

143 *list of myths*: This list is adapted, edited, and expanded from American Hospice Foundation, "Debunking the Myths of Hospice," and from "Learning about Hospice," Americanhospice.org.

143 *local community nonprofits*: Long-standing nonprofit hospices often have good reputations, but keep an open mind: some for-profit hospices do an excellent job.

144 *life-extending rather than palliative*: As of 2017, a few Medicare pilot programs allow people to get curative treatment and limited hospice benefits at the same time—another program I think should be expanded. (To my mind, anybody within about eighteen months of dying should have the right to medical care at home, whether it is called

"home-based palliative care," "serious illness management," or "hospice.")

145 *lasting up to an hour or so*: Medicare reimburses hospices at a higher rate for "continuous care" at the bedside or in a separate residential hospice for a few days if a patient's symptoms become unmanageable or caregivers need respite. In practice, this respite is usually short term and rare. Ask for it if you need it.

148 *Ask around about friends' experience*: "Hospice Compare" on the Medicare website lets you get a list of hospices serving your zip code and compare their ratings. Questions for your first one-to-one meeting, suggested by Hospice Foundation of America, are listed in the resource section.

150 *rancher Jim Modini*: The Modinis' end of life story was told by their neighbor Judy MacDonald Johnston in her excellent TED Talk "Prepare for a Good End of Life."

152 *microbiologist Louis Pasteur*: Michael Stolberg, *A History of Palliative Care, 1500–1970: Concepts, Practices, and Ethical Challenges* (Springer, 2017), p. 129.

152 *novelist Léon Daudet*: *Devant La Douleur* (1915), pp. 62–63, translation by Katy Butler. CF. Stolberg.

153 *support for expanding*: For more information on physician-assisted dying, contact Compassion and Choices (compassionandchoices.org).

153 *Greek philosopher Cleanthes*: Jerry B. Wilson, *Death by Decision* (Westminster Press, 1975), p. 22. Citing W. Mair, "Suicide: Greek and Roman," *Encyclopedia of Religion and Ethics*, 1925.

154 *chose to stop eating and drinking*: See Phyllis Shacter, "Choosing to Die: A Personal Story. Elective Death by Voluntarily Stopping Eating and Drinking (VSED) in the Face of Degenerative Disease." CreateSpace Independent Publishing Platform, 2017.

154 *After spending his last week*: See Derek Humphry, *Final Exit: The Practicalities of Self-Deliverance and Assisted Suicide for the Dying* (First published in 1991; Bantam Dell, 2010).

154 *Phillip's wife, Aida*: Aida and Phillip's names have been changed.

156 "*Goodbye*": Ira Byock, *The Four Things That Matter Most* (Atria Books, 2014).

158 *handbook*: Cappy Capossela and Sheila Warnock, *Share the Care: How to Organize a Group to Care for Someone Who Is Seriously Ill* (Touchstone, 2004). See Sharethecare.org.

CHAPTER 7: *Active Dying*

162 Late Fragment: Raymond Carver, "Late Fragment," from *A New Path to the Waterfall* (Atlantic Monthly Press, 1989). Reprinted by permission.

165 *named Gordon*: Names and some identifying details have been changed.

171 *a bone marrow transplant*: "Stem Cell Transplant for Multiple Myeloma," American Cancer Society website. https://www.cancer.org/cancer/multiple-myeloma/treating/stem-cell-transplant.html. Accessed January 8, 2017.

171 *could kill him*: Between 41 and 60 percent of people receiving bone marrow from another person die within the first year. See Memorial Sloan Kettering, "MSK's One-Year Survival Rate after Allogenic Bone Marrow Transplant Exceeds Expectations," online press release, March 26, 2012, https://www.mskcc.org/blog/msk-s-one-year-survival-rate-after-allogenic-bone-marrow-transplant-exceeds-expectations. Accessed January 10, 2018. Federally mandated survival statistics, by transplant center, are listed in the Transplant Center Directory, at Bethematch.org, accessed January 12, 2018.

172 *morally responsible institutional culture*: E. Dzeng, et al., "Influence of Institutional Culture and Policies on Do-Not-Resuscitate Decision Making at the End of Life," *JAMA Internal Medicine* 175, no. 5 (May 2015):812–819. doi: 10.1001/jamainternmed.2015.0295. Accessed Feb 9, 2018.

172 *"Buddhist perspective"*: The notion that suffering is redemptive is not in fact a teaching of classical Buddhism, which holds that suffering results from not accepting things as they are.

174 *To keep him from developing bedsores*: Hospice nurses recommend turning every two to four hours, and less frequently when death is very near. Many people find cleaning the bottoms and changing the diapers of close family members—especially a parent or sibling—repellent. Anne had thirty years of practice as a nurse, and she approached the task matter-of-factly, and as an act of love. Not everyone can. "It's important," she said, "for people to honor their limitations. There is no shame in hiring an aide for these very difficult jobs."

183 *has been dead for hours*: I recommend this explicit language to avoid traumatic attempts at CPR.

183 *a chain of circumstances*: In New York City and many other places, paramedics have performed CPR for as long as forty minutes, even when the person has been dead for more than an hour and family members plead that CPR be halted.

184 *writing mentor Barry*: Barry is a pseudonym.

184 *Liz wrote on her blog*: Liz Salmi, "Hacking the Hospital Death," the lizarmy.com. April 30, 2016. Adapted with permission.

186 *as the RESPECT protocol*: RESPECT stands for: Restore order, Explain what happened, Stop other duties; be Present, Empathize, offer to call a Chaplain for spiritual support, and allow the family Time with the dead or dying person.

190 *ritually wash the body*: Debra Rodgers first learned about bathing rituals at a Metta Institute workshop for medical professionals led by

Frank Ostaseski, a cofounder of San Francisco Zen Hospice, and author of *Five Invitations: Discovering What Death Can Teach Us About Living Fully.* Flatiron, March 2017.

CONCLUSION: *Toward a New Art of Dying*

198 *death in the abstract*: For this insight I am indebted to Bart Windrum, author of *Happy Landings: A Gateway to Peaceful Dying.*

199 *pathway to a good death*: PACE (Program for All Inclusive Care of the Elderly) is free to people on Medicaid who are over age fifty-five, need significant help with practical daily activities, and can, with support, live outside nursing homes (either with relatives, in assisted living, or on their own). It is only available in some areas.

People on Medicare can join PACE by paying the equivalent of their monthly Medicare premium, plus about $700 to $1,000 per month for prescription drug coverage. That sounds like a breathtaking amount, but it may be cheaper and less time-consuming (and much more fun and healthy for the frail elder) than full-time home care, assisted living, a nursing home, or a patchwork of private services. To see if there's a program in your area, check the website of the National PACE association at npaonline.org.

GLOSSARY

218 *Short-term survival rates*: Brady, K. K. Gurka, B. Mehring, et al., "In-hospital cardiac arrest: Impact of monitoring and witnessed event on patient survival and neurologic status at hospital discharge," *Resuscitation*, no. 82 (2011):845–852.

223 *Overdiagnosis*: For guidance on this and several other glossary entries, I am indebted to Slow Medicine (Italia) and its *Le Parole della medicina che cambia: Un dizionario critico.* Ill Pensiero Scientifico Editore, May 2017.

Acknowledgments

This book started out as a slim volume of aphorisms and self-help tips. I quickly learned that if it were to find its true shape, I would need to include the stories, experience, and wisdom of people who knew more than I did. The following people, and others whom I have not named, taught me that dying well is rarely done alone. It takes a village, and so has writing this book. My gratitude is boundless.

Many people shared personal stories about aging, illness, and good and difficult deaths. I was moved, enlightened, and changed by Jackie Adams, Kelcy Allwein, Jennifer Moore Ballentine, Amy Berman, the late Merijane Block, Diana C., the late Mary Jane Denzer, Bronni Galin, Judy MacDonald Johnston, Laura Lamar, Robert Levering, Anne Masterson, RN, Sharry Mullin, Cathryn Ramin, Karen Randall, Ed R., Liz Salmi, Jane Sidwell, Amy Sousa, Doug von Koss, Leslie Walker, and the late Mary Wolfe. Thank you for helping me understand more, and fear less. I also thank people whom I cannot name. You know who you are.

Members of the Facebook group Slow Medicine responded to random questions when only a family caregiver, medical advocate, physical therapist, speech therapist, occupational therapist, hospice nurse, or palliative care doctor could help me. Thank you to all of you, and especially those who vetted individual chapters, including Katie Armatruda; Alisha Benner, MD; Lisa Berry

Blackstock; Toby Brandtman, MD; Patti Bartholomew Heaps, RN; Christine Khandelwal, OD; Amy Lustig, SLT; Mary Anne Miller, RN; Mary-Jean Paulitz, PT; Lori Perrine, RN; Ellen Schweigert; and Jerry Soucy, RN. Any errors that remain are my own.

Gratitude is due to all hospice workers, activists, doctors, insurers, nurses, and researchers passionate about improving the American experience of the end of life. Those who deepened my understanding include Megory Anderson, D.Th., Robert Arnold, MD, Anthony Back, MD, Amy Berman and our colleagues at Carelab, Atul Gawande, MD, Valery Hazanov, PhD, Shoshana Helman, MD, Daniel Hoefer, MD, Redwing Keyssar, RN, Joanne Lynn, MD, Diana Meier, MD, the late Dennis McCullough, MD, BJ Miller, MD, Susan Mitchell, MD, Siddhartha Mukherjee, MD, Sunita Puri, MD, Debra Rodgers, RN, Phyllis Shacter, Victoria Sweet, MD, Joan Teno, MD, Jessica Nutik Zitter, MD, Dawn Gross, MD, Thomas J. Smith, MD, Judy Thomas, JD at the Coalition for Compassionate Care of California, Eric Widera, MD, and Bart Windrum. Thank you.

The poet Jane Hirshfield, in a spontaneous act of friendship, read and commented on the entire manuscript at a late stage. My thanks to Jane, and to my delightful and skilled writing partners Anne Cushman and Katherine Ellison, who read drafts of many chapters. My gratitude extends beyond them to Jonathan Butler, Zoe Carter, Jonathan Dann, Susan Ito, Eva Shoshany, and to members of my former writing group: Molly Giles, Laura Hilgers, Jonathan Krim, and Stefanie Marlis.

In a rapidly changing literary landscape, I am honored to call Amanda Urban my literary agent, and Scribner my publisher. Thank you to Kara Watson for her delicate editing, and to Abigail Novak, Dani Spencer, Nan Graham, Susan Moldow, Brian Belfiglio, and Roz Lippel, for helping this book find its readers and its home. Thank you for believing in me.

For research and other forms of invaluable professional help,

I thank Constance Hale, Leslie Jackson, Joy Johannessen, Leslie Keenan, Mary Ladd, Elizabeth Savage, Rebecca Sheranian, and Rebecca Snyder. Special thanks are due to Leah Rosenbaum and to Joanna Czerny, my lecture agent, for keeping me out of the weeds and helping me to spread the word.

I was blessed with the gift of uninterrupted writing time, in beautiful surroundings, at Mesa Refuge in Point Reyes, California, and at the Corporation of Yaddo in Saratoga Springs, New York. Thank you to the philanthropists and visionaries who support artists and writers. You make much beauty possible.

Finally, I am grateful daily for my husband, Brian Donohue, who listened to every chapter read aloud and keeps teaching me how to find the joy in any situation.

Permissions

Index

acupuncture, 99, 217
ADLs (activities of daily living), 55, 213
advance directives (ADs), 24, 28, 214
  comfort measures on, 119, 126–29, 133, 192, 217, 229
  dementia and, 119–21, 129, 133
  as legal right, 26
  multiple backup copies of, 119
  obtaining forms for, 28, 33–34
advanced illness, 77, 214
"against medical advice" (AMA) discharge from hospitals, 116, 131
aging
  developmental tasks related to, 31
  health stages of later life and, 8
  medical risks with, 21
  people's acceptance of, 6–7
  Slowing Down health stage and, 40
Alberts, Alan, 153–54
Alcoholics Anonymous, 20, 33, 237
alcohol use, and lifestyle changes, 16
allow natural death (AND) orders, 120, 128, 133, 218, 219
alternative medicine, 217
Alzheimer's Association, 86, 124
American Academy of Home Care Medicine, 119

American Board of Internal Medicine (ABIM), 49, 227, 235
American Cancer Society, 86, 235
American Geriatrics Society, "Beers List" from, 52, 214, 240
American Heart Association, 91
American Society of Clinical Oncology, 91
ancillary health care workers, 60
AND (allow natural death) orders, 120, 128, 133, 218, 219
anticholinergics, 39, 47, 48, 52, 214, 239
Ars Moriendi (medieval text), 3–4
aspirin, 47, 99
assisted living residences
  Adaptation health stage and, 55, 61
  cost of, 57, 62, 68, 166
  frailty and, 107
  response to medical events in, 113, 118
attending physician, 214–15

Back, Anthony, 83, 93–94, 98, 100
back surgery, 21
balance
  exercise programs for, 16, 65
  medications affecting, 39, 40, 46
Beacon Hill Village, 58

"Beers List" (American Geriatrics Society), 52, 214, 240
Being Mortal (Gawande), 7, 86
benzodiazepines, 47–48, 146, 240
Berman, Amy, 78–81, 84, 92, 95, 102–3
bioethics committee, 215
blood pressure
  lifestyle changes to lower, 19, 20
  medications for, 19, 20, 33, 38, 46, 74, 115, 129
Bourne, Molly, 147–48
brain
  medications harming, 46, 47, 52
  See also cognitive abilities
Buddhism, 32, 170, 182

Calmes, Beth, 190
cancer
  diet in treatment of, 99
  drugs for, 94
  hospice for, 146–47
  immunotherapy for, 95
  medical marijuana for, 99–100
  online sources for, 86, 235
  stage four, 77, 84, 85, 141, 147, 164, 228
  strengthening immune system in, 99
  survival times in, 94, 95
capacity, 215
cardiac catheterization, 110
cardiac defibrillators, implanted, 124, 130, 133
cardiac rehabilitation programs, 15
cardiac surgery, 109, 110
cardiopulmonary resuscitation (CPR), 217–18
  care decisions on, 124
  do-not-resuscitate (DNR) orders covering, 120, 218
  POLSTs and MOLSTs on, 119, 120, 218
care, definition of, 215

caregivers
  alliance for, 236
  community programs for older people with respite for, 71
  complex relationship with, 72
  death's impact on, 142
  dementia and, 107, 114, 122, 124
  dilemma of when to stop medical procedures, 122
  dying process and, 168, 169, 232
  finding and hiring, 71
  frail people and, 112–13, 129
  home death and, 176–77, 178
  hospice and, 144, 147–48
  online discussion group for, 237–38
  PACE support for, 199
  paid home care to help, 69, 70, 74
  POLST and, 119, 121
  terminal illness and, 70, 74, 85
caregiving role
  family and, 70, 74, 236
  tribe for sharing, 23, 158
C. diff infection, 139
charge nurses, 215
chemo brain, 216
chemotherapy
  financial incentives for using, 96
  quality of life and, 99
cholesterol-lowering statins, 18, 46, 74
Choosing to Die (Shacter), 154, 233
Choosing Wisely website, 49, 52, 227, 235
chronic illness, 77, 216
circling the drain, 216, 220
clinical effectiveness, 216
clinical trials, 97–98
coding, 216
cognitive abilities
  Adaptation health stage and, 63
  annual assessments of, 20
  cholesterol-lowering statins affecting, 46

post-operative decline of, 22, 225
prednisone and other steroids
    affecting, 48
sleep drugs affecting, 240
Slowing Down health stage and,
    37
cognitive reserve, 45
Cologuard screening tests, 49
colonoscopies, 49
comfort care, 68, 91, 145, 164,
    216–17
    dementia and, 126–29, 133
    sample letter on, 127–29
comfort measures, orders for, 119,
    126–29, 133, 192, 217, 229
community support programs
    and services, 60, 62, 70–71,
    236–38
complementary medicine, 99, 217
concierge practices, 44–45
congestive heart failure (CHF), 217
Conversation Project, 28, 33, 240
CPR. *See* cardiopulmonary
    resuscitation
crash carts, 218
Cruzan, Nancy, 26–27
Cunningham nursing home, 204–5
cyanosis, 218

daily life
    disaster-proofing your home
        against risks in, 64–67
    simplifying, in Slowing Down
        health stage, 41, 52
DASH (Doctors Assisting Seniors
    at Home), Santa Barbara,
    California, 117–18
death and dying, 1–9, 161–93, 218
    Ars Moriendi (medieval text) on,
        3–4
    behavior of gravely ill person
        before, 163
    care provided during, 180–81
    ceremonies of death and, 182

choosing time of, 152–55
desire to reclaim power to shape
    experience of, 5
emotional legacy after, 156–57
final hours in, 182–83
five emotional tasks before, 156,
    160
goodbye rituals in, 190–91
"good death" concept and, 29, 30,
    33, 168, 197–98, 205
health stages of later life and, 8
hoping to die well, 3
hospital and medical technologies
    signs of, 164
hospital setting for, 5–6, 7,
    184–90, 192
life support removal before, 164,
    184, 224
making use of time left before,
    138–39
medical rights and planning ahead
    for, 24
notifications to be made after, 183
people's feelings and wishes
    about, 7, 9
physical process of, 168–69,
    175–76
physician-assisted, 152–53, 214,
    219, 222, 226
poem and prayer recitations
    during, 192–93
preparing for, 135–60
reform movement focused on,
    7–8
settling affairs before, 149–51
story about new art of, 197–209
story about signs before, 165–68
support circle for, 158–59, 160
ways to prepare for, 160, 192
47, 65, 74
See also dying at home
Death Cafes, 7
defibrillators, 218
    implanted, 124, 130, 133

dementia, 107–33, 218
  advance directives for, 119–21
  care during last years of, 129–32
  caregivers' dilemma over
      prolonging life in, 122–24
  comfort care in, 126–29, 133
  coping with, 122–24
  goal of treatment in, 111–12
  house call programs in, 116–19
  medications causing, 47, 52
  precarious health in, 111
  resources for, 124
  statements describing, 107
  stories of families dealing with,
      124–26, 130–32
  as terminal illness, 121–22
  trajectory in, 112, 122
  ways to prepare for, 133
Devine, Meghan, 112
diabetes, 16, 18–19, 129
diabetes prevention programs, 20,
    33, 43, 46
diet
  cardiac health and, 15, 19
  diabetes and, 18, 19
  last years in dementia and, 129,
    133
  life-limiting illnesses and, 99, 101
  lifestyle changes affecting, 16, 19
DNR orders. See do-not-resuscitate
    (DNR) orders
doctors
  Adaptation health stage and
      overall health assessment
      from, 61
  financial incentives for using
      medications and, 43, 96
  frailty as distinct health stage and,
    113
  goals of care and, 77, 96, 164, 203,
    221
  health maintenance organizations
      (HMOs) and, 43
  overmedication and, 45–46

preventive medicine and, 20, 33
  referrals for physical, speech, or
      occupational therapy from,
      63, 74
  retirement communities with, 68
  talking about terminal illness
      diagnoses with, 83–85, 94,
      104
  training in talking about terminal
      illness for, 83, 94
  See also geriatricians; primary
      care doctors
Dolara, Alberto, 42
do not hospitalize (DNH), 218
do-not-resuscitate (DNR) orders, 28,
    120–21, 133, 192, 218, 219
  home death and, 178
  keeping multiple backup copies
      of, 119, 121
  Medic Alert bracelet for, 121, 127,
      178
  possible ignoring of, 121
do not transport (DNT), 218
drinking
  alcohol use and lifestyle changes,
      16, 20, 33, 237
  voluntary stopping of eating and
      drinking (VSED), 153, 154,
      178, 180, 206, 229
  water intake and, 37, 65, 115
driving, decision to stop, 55, 56, 67
drugs. See medications
Drugs.com, 46, 235
Dunn, Hank, 124, 232
durable power of attorney for health
    care, 28, 33, 225
  choosing ideal person as, 28, 33
  See also power of attorney (POA)
Dwindles trajectory, 86, 89, 112
dying. See death and dying
dying at home
  Americans' desire for, 5
  earlier family experience with, 4
  hospice nurse and, 174, 175–76

Medicare Advantage plans and, 44
preparing for, 176–79
story about, 170–76
ways to prepare for, 192

eating
lifestyle changes affecting, 16, 19
voluntary stopping of eating and
drinking (VSED), 153, 154,
178, 180, 206, 229
See also diet
edema, 219
Eden Alternative, 204
Ehrenreich, Barbara, 7
Emanuel, Ezekiel, 44
emesis, 219
end stage illness, 77, 219
euthanasia, 219, 224
evidence-based medicine (EBM), 43,
219–20, 235
exercise
aging and maintaining
functioning using, 15–16, 17,
18, 19, 33, 40, 99, 129
overcoming challenges in, 19
pain management and, 46, 47
rehabilitation and, 63, 64, 72
sleep and, 48

failed back surgery syndrome, 21
failure to thrive, 220
fall prevention classes, 43, 65, 74
falls
aging bodies and, 16, 65
causes of, 114–15
exercise to prevent, 64–65, 74
eyesight and, 65
fire department's "Lift and Assist"
service for, 114
frailty and, 107, 108, 113, 114–15
during hospital stays, 109
house assessment for, 65–66, 241
medications and risk for, 45, 46,
47, 48, 50, 52, 129, 239, 240

retirement community policies
on, 68
family
caregiving role and, 70, 74
conversations about medical
decisions with, 29–30
legacy letters to, 100
morphine prescriptions and fears
of, 145–46, 174, 177
terminal illness and, 89–90,
102–3
Final Exit Network, 154
financial plans
Adaptation health stage and, 62,
74
death and, 102
hospice and, 143
Medicaid and, 62–63, 66, 70, 241
FIT screening tests, 49
"Five Wishes" advance directive,
28, 33
Fonda, Jane, exercise videos from,
64, 238
Food and Drug Administration
(FDA), 21, 94, 98
fragility, 220
frailty, 107
advance directives in, 119–21
factors in hospitalization decision
for, 114–16
hospitalization's impact on,
109–11, 113–14
house call programs in, 116–19
"House of Cards" health stage,
111–112, 124, 129
recognizing as distinct health
stage, 112–13
possible services needed by,
112–13
statements describing, 107
story about family's approach to,
108–10
surgery decisions in, 115–16
frequent flyers, 114, 221

friends
  acceptance of reality of death by,
    29–30
  bad diagnoses and support from,
    82, 83, 84
  conversations about medical
    decisions with, 29–30
  disability and help from, 69, 74
  dying at home and, 177, 178, 179,
    182
  dying in a hospital and, 184–85,
    186, 189–90
  exercising with, 18
  hospice and, 144, 145, 148
  making a move and finding, 67, 68
  neighbors as, 22–24, 33, 69
  preparing for death and, 143, 154,
    158, 159
  as proxies or health care agents,
    28, 30, 33
  retirement communities and, 68
  support networks with, 23, 57, 60,
    69–70, 142, 160
  surgery support from, 116
  as a tribe, 23, 24, 158–59, 176
  younger people as, 22, 33, 69
funeral plans, 102, 137, 174, 199,
  208

Galin, Bronni, 56–59
Gawande, Atul, 7, 83, 86, 212
geriatricians, 52, 211, 221
  goal of, 114
  medication reviews by, 39, 45–46,
    129, 130
  preventive medicine and, 20
  screenings and, 49
geriatrics, 8, 238
  pharmacists with specialized
    knowledge of, 45–46
  Slowing Down health stage and,
    41
goals of care, 77, 96, 164, 203, 221

GoGo Grandparent rider service, 58
Gross, Dawn, 93

Hard Choices for Loving People
  (Dunn), 124, 232
Hazanov, Valery, 72–73
health care agent or health care
  advocate, 28, 85, 122, 158, 215,
  225, 226
health care system
  Adaptation health stage and, 60
  concierge practices and, 44–45
  reform movement focused on
    dying and, 8
  Slow Medicine movement and, 42
health insurance
  hospices and, 145
  house call programs and, 118
  Medicare Advantage plans and,
    42–43, 43–44, 52, 117, 240–41
  obtaining medical rights forms
    from, 28
  wellness appointments under, 20
health maintenance organizations
  (HMOs), 42–43, 44, 52, 67,
  115, 240–41
health screenings, 41, 49, 52, 223,
  227, 235
Heiser, K. Gabriel, 63, 241
Helman, Shoshana, 100
high-value care, 221
Hippocratic oath, 26, 27, 152
HMOs (health maintenance
  organizations), 42–43, 44, 52,
  67, 115, 240–41
Hoefer, Daniel, 48, 108, 109
Hoffman, Ron, 84
Home Based Primary Care
  program (HBPC), Veterans
  Administration, 116, 242
home death. *See* dying at home
home health aides, 58, 62, 69, 71–72,
  145, 200, 225, 238

hope, in terminal illness, 7, 82, 84, 100–102
hospice, 2–3, 143–49, 221–22
  Medicare Advantage plans and, 44
  morphine and other medications used in, 145–46
  myths about, 143–48
  next steps in learning about, 148–49
  researching options in, 148
  story about, 170–76
  talking with doctors about, 83, 104
hospice nurses, and dying at home, 174, 175–76
hospital delirium, 222
hospitalization
  factors in decision for frail people's stay of, 114–16
  Medicare Advantage plans and rates of, 44
hospitals
  cardiac rehabilitation programs in, 15
  frail people's reactions to stays in, 109–11, 113–14
  leaving "against medical advice" (AMA), 116, 131
  as setting for dying, 5–6, 7, 184–90, 192
house call programs, 116–19, 145, 148, 179
housing
  Adaptation health stage and choices in, 58–59, 67–69
  disaster-proofing against risks in, 64–67
How to Protect Your Family's Assets from Devastating Nursing Home Costs (Heiser), 63, 241

IADLs (instrumental activities of daily living). *See* ADLs (activities of daily living)

immune system
  aging and, 40
  bone marrow transplantation in cancer and, 171
  C. diff infection in hospitals and, 139
  impact of trauma to, 108
  medications weakening, 48
  radiation therapy in cancer and, 92
  strengthening of, in cancer treatment, 99
immunotherapy, 95
implanted cardiac devices (ICDs). *See* defibrillators; pacemakers
incurable illness, 77, 81, 222
Institute of Medicine, 209
instrumental activities of daily living (IADLs). *See* ADLs (activities of daily living)
insurance. *See* health insurance
intensive care units (ICUs), 44, 121, 149, 164, 184–85, 189
  deaths in, 5

Johnston, Judy MacDonald, 24, 237

Kaiser Permanente systems, 43, 44, 186, 210, 240
Kalanithi, Paul, 7
Keyssar, Judith Redwing, 155, 188

Lamar, Laura, and "Marj," 38–40
late-stage illness, 77
law of double effect, 222
legacy letters, 100
lifestyle, changes in, 16–17, 20, 40, 217
life support, removal of, 164, 184, 224
living wills, 24, 27, 214
  areas covered in, 28
  obtaining forms for, 28
  See also advance directives (ADs)

loneliness, 22, 70
Looping Decline trajectory, 86,
    87–88
Loretto programs, 199, 204
loss, making peace with, 50–51, 52
Lovelace, Ada, 99–100
Lustig, Amy, 44
Lynn, Joanne, 86

marijuana, medical use of, 99–100
Marin Villages, 58, 241
Maynard, Brittany, 152–53
Mayo Clinic, 86, 235
McCullough, Dennis, 42, 232
Meals on Wheels, 60, 112–13, 236
Medicaid
    bedside care near death and, 158
    finances and qualifying for, 62–63,
        66, 69, 70, 199, 241
    home health aides under, 62
    hospice and, 145
    nursing home care under, 62
    website for, 237
medical aid in dying (MIA), 222
medical care
    Adaptation health stage and, 60
    frailty as distinct health stage and,
        112–13
Medic Alert Foundation, 121, 127, 178
medical orders for life-sustaining
    treatment. See MOLST
    (medical orders for life-
    sustaining treatment)
medical power of attorney, 28, 33,
    225, 226
medical rights, 24–30
    conversations with family and
        friends about, 29–30
    Cruzan decision and, 26–27
    examples of, 28
    obtaining forms for, 28–29
    sending copies of forms to
        physicians, 30

medical risks, evaluating, 21–22
Medicare, 211
    choosing authorized
        representative for, 33
    hospice benefit under, 144–45,
        147, 148
    house call programs and, 118,
        145
    Medicare Advantage plans
        compared with, 44
    physical therapy under, 63–64
    skilled nursing facility (SKF)
        under, 144–45, 166
    taking advantage of coverage
        under, 21
    wellness appointments under, 20
Medicare Advantage health plans,
    42–43, 43–44, 52, 117,
    240–41
medication reviews, 39, 45–46, 129,
    130
medications
    clinical trials of, 97–98
    financial incentives for using, 43,
        96
    health maintenance organizations
        (HMOs) and, 43
    hospices and, 146
    overmedication and, 45–46
    periodic reviews of, 39, 45–46,
        129, 130
medicine
    evidence-based, 43, 219–20, 235
    hospitals as setting for dying and,
        5–6
    prevention and, 20–21, 33
    prolonging life of body as mission
        of, 6
    Slowing Down health stage and
        expectations of, 41
    Slow Medicine approach to, 8, 42,
        228, 234, 237–38
Mediterranean diet, 15, 99

melatonin, 48
memory
    Adaptation health stage and, 61,
        72
    dementia and, 119–21, 129, 133
    hospital stays and, 110, 222
    keeping multiple backup copies
        of, 119
    MOLST (medical orders for life-
        sustaining treatment), 28, 223
    prednisone and other steroids
        affecting, 48
    Slowing Down health stage and,
        40
    walking and increase in, 17
mood distress, 223
morphine, 140, 145–46, 174, 177,
    181, 217
Moss, Alvin H. "Woody," 83, 84
mourning rituals, 31, 51, 102–3
Mukherjee, Siddhartha, 98, 99
multiple co-morbidities, 223
multiple organ systems failure, 223
Murphy, Tom, 18
Mydirectives.com, 28, 33

National Suicide Prevention hotline,
    155
Natural Causes (Ehrenreich), 7
neighbors
    friendships with, 22–24, 33
    support network with, 69
Niagara Falls trajectory, 86–87
Norman, John and Philippa 1–2
nosocomial conditions, 223
nursing homes
    Eden Alternative in, 204
    Gordon Lechenger, death in,
        165–68
    Loretta Downs, creation of
        "Chrysalis Rooms," 179
    Manfreddi family, experience with
        death in, 197–209

    Medicaid coverage of, 62
    preparing for dying in, 179–80

occupational therapy, 8, 60, 63,
    65–66, 74, 91, 117, 199, 210
Oliver, Mary, 153
open-heart surgery, 22, 109
opiates, 146
O'Reilly, Matthew, 149
overdiagnosis, 223
overmedication, 45–46, 48
overtreatment, 224
    dementia and, 132
    overdiagnosis leading to, 223
    Slow Medicine and, 42

PACE (Program of All-Inclusive
    Care for the Elderly), 198–202,
    203, 204–5, 208, 209, 210
pacemakers, 2, 224
painkillers
    advance directives on, 119, 128
    from drugstores, 46–47
pain management, 21, 46, 91, 144,
    146, 158, 167, 186, 192, 224
palliative care, 224
    benefits of, 91
    decision on when to begin, 93
    terminal illness with, 90–92, 93,
        104
palliative care doctors, 86, 90, 92, 97,
    104, 139, 215
Pap tests, 49
patient representative, 225
patient-centered care, 8, 225
Perrine, Lori, 188
person-centered care, 21, 225
pharmaceutical industry
    financial incentives for, 96
    information website funding by,
        86
pharmacists, medication reviews by,
    45–46

physical therapy, 8, 20, 18, 60,
    63–64, 74, 91, 117, 129, 143,
    200, 210, 211
  adaptation health stage and, 60
  pain management with, 47
  physician referrals to, 20, 74
physician-assisted suicide, 152–53,
    214, 219, 222, 226
physician orders, 225. *See also
    specific orders*
physician orders for life-sustaining
    treatment. *See* POLST
    (physician orders for life-
    sustaining treatment)
physicians. *See* doctors
Physician's Desk Reference, 46, 233
Pilates, 64, 65, 74
podiatrists, 18, 200
POLST (physician orders for life-
    sustaining treatment), 28, 218,
    225
  dementia and, 119–21, 129, 133
  keeping multiple backup copies
    of, 119
post-operative cognitive decline
    (POCD), 22, 225
power of attorney (POA), 225.
    See also durable power of
    attorney
prednisone, 47
prescription medications. *See*
    medications
preventive medicine, 20–21, 33
primary care doctors, 226
  concierge practices and, 44–45
  establishing rapport with, 20–21
  finding a younger doctor for, 20
  medical decision documents sent
    to, 30
  medication reviews by, 45–46
  preventive medicine and, 20, 33
  Slow Medicine movement and,
    42
prognosis, 226

progressive illness, 77, 226
proxy, 28, 33, 215, 226
PSA (prostate cancer) tests, 49, 223

quality of life, 226
  chemotherapy and, 99
  medicine's goals for, 6
  people's survey responses on, 7

refusal of medical treatment, legal
    right to, 26, 27
religious beliefs
  contemplation of death and,
    31–32
  medical technologies in
    prolonging life and, 123–24
religious groups, retirement
    communities of, 68–69
response rate, 227
retirement communities, questions
    to ask when choosing, 67–69
risk management, 227
Royal Canadian Air Force exercise,
    64, 129

Schultz, Zacharias, 9
screenings, 41, 49, 52, 223, 227, 235
sepsis, 227
Shacter, Phyllis, 154, 233
shared medical decision-making,
    227–28
Share the Care (Caposella and
    Warnock), 158, 242
simplifying
  Adaptation health stage and,
    61–62
  Slowing Down health stage and,
    41, 52
skilled nursing facility (SNF), 109,
    144–45, 166, 228
sleep
  exercise and, 16
  fixes for problems with, 48
sleeping pills, 39, 47–48, 74, 214

Slow Medicine, 8, 42, 228, 234,
    237–38
smoking, and lifestyle changes, 16,
    17, 20, 33, 237
speech therapy, 44, 63, 74
spirituality, 31–32
    contemplation of death and,
        31–32, 33
    nursing home residents and, 73
stage four cancer, 77, 84, 85, 141,
    147, 164, 228
stair step down trajectory, 86, 88,
    112
statins, 18, 46, 74
steroids, 47
Stolberg, Michael, 25
strength
    aging and changes in, 89
    ways of improving, 65, 99
strength training, 15–16, 239
suicide
    hotline for, 155
    physician-assisted, 152–53, 214,
        219, 222, 226
support groups, 20, 33, 43, 83, 97,
    104, 237
support networks, 23, 57, 60, 69–70,
    142
    death preparations and, 158–59,
        160
support programs and services, 60,
    62, 236
surgery
    cognitive decline after, 22, 225
    frail people and, 115–16
    medical risks in, 22
surrogate, 33, 215, 225, 226
    choosing ideal person as, 28, 33
    obtaining forms for, 28
surrogate effectiveness, 227, 228

t'ai chi, 64, 65, 74
terminal illness, 220, 222, 228
    clinical trials during, 97–98

death-hastening prescriptions
    and, 152, 214, 219, 222
dementia as, 121–22
doctor's diagnosis of, 77, 84, 137
enjoying time left in, 100–102
fears about, 94
hope in, 7, 82, 84, 100–102
hospice for, 143, 181
online sources for, 86, 235
palliative care in, 90–92, 93
patient's focus on family in, 102–3
patient's staying in charge during,
    94–97
preparing family for, 89–90
story about patient handling
    diagnosis of, 78–81
support groups for, 83
support programs for, 237
treatment for, 95, 146
understanding trajectory of, 85–89
what life activities matter to
    patient during, 93–94
terminal sedation, 228
Total palliative sedation, 228
tribe, friends as, 23, 24, 158–59, 176
Tylenol, 46, 47

Uber, 58

Veterans Administration, 116, 242
Villages mutual aid network, 58, 67,
    237, 241
visiting nurse programs, 117, 119
Visiting Physicians Associations,
    118, 119, 242
Vitaltalk, 83, 94
voluntary stopping of eating and
    drinking (VSED), 153, 154,
    178, 180, 206, 229
Von Koss, Doug, 14, 16, 21, 24, 50,
    67

Walski, Ed, 124–26
walkers, 39, 55, 63, 66–67, 107, 108

walking
    Alzheimer's and, 147, 148
    benefits of, 17–18
    cane for, 64
    dementia and, 122
    frailty and, 107
    hospitalization and, 110, 111, 115
water
    staying hydrated, 37, 65, 115
    voluntary stopping of, 203, 229

water-walking, 37, 56, 58
ways to prepare suggestions, 33, 52,
    74, 104, 133, 160, 192
wellness appointments, 20–21
When Breath Becomes Air
    (Kalanithi), 7
Widera, Eric, 46, 115

yoga, 47, 65, 74